Curriculum Development from a Nursing Model

MARGUERITE B. WHITE has a B.S. from Skidmore College, M.S. from Syracuse University, and Ed.D. from Teachers College, Columbia University. She is Professor Emeritus at the University of Connecticut. During the development and implementation of this curriculum, she was Associate Dean in charge of the undergraduate program at the University of Connecticut and, for three years, curriculum project director. Dr. White has also taught at Skidmore College, Syracuse University, and Wagner College.

Curriculum Development from a Nursing Model

The Crisis Theory Framework

Marguerite B. White, Ed.D.

Editor

Springer Publishing Company/New York

Springer Publishing Company, Inc.
200 Park Avenue South
New York, New York 10003

83 84 85 86 87 / 10 9 8 7 6 5 4 3 2 1

Library of Congress Cataloging in Publication Data
Main entry under title:

Curriculum development from a nursing model.
  (Springer series on the teaching of nursing ; v. 8)
  Bibliography: p.
  Includes index.
  1. Nursing—Study and teaching—Philosophy—Addresses, essays, lectures. 2. Curriculum planning—Addresses, essays, lectures. I. White, Marguerite B. II. Series. [DNLM: 1. Education, Nursing. 2. Curriculum. 3. Models, Theoretical. W1 SP685Sg v.8 / WY 18 C9745]
RT73.C874 1983   610.73'07'11   83-4758
ISBN 0-8261-3280-4

Printed in the United States of America

Contents

Preface

This book is an outgrowth of an extensive curriculum revision initiated in 1968 by the faculty of the University of Connecticut School of Nursing. Although the existing curriculum had been adequate in the fifties and sixties, the faculty no longer believed that it was preparing the type of professional practitioner that would be needed in the future. Changes in nurse practice acts and in society's expectations for health care mandated changes in educational programs. The trend toward greater independence in nursing practice required better preparation for responsible decision making. With increasing emphasis on health maintenance and community-based practice, additional theoretical content as well as additional tools and techniques for client assessment were needed.

Moreover, the existing curriculum pattern involved considerable duplication of content and fostered compartmentalization of knowledge rather than integration. These factors, together with the tremendous increase in scientific knowledge relevant to nursing, made it increasingly difficult to include the essential content. The problem was compounded by the absence of a clearly defined conceptual framework to guide the selection and organization of content and learning experiences. The outcome of initial faculty efforts toward change was the writing and subsequent funding by the Division of Nursing, Department of Health, Education, and Welfare of a five-year curriculum project to strengthen the baccalaureate nursing program at the University of Connecticut by developing a curriculum based on a theoretical approach to nursing content.

In the late 1960s and early 1970s, the University of Connecticut faculty was relatively inexperienced in curriculum construction. Some faculty had a dream of a unique nursing curriculum based on a nursing model rather than a medical model, but very few faculty members really understood the meaning of a nursing model or a conceptual framework. Since the early 1960s, theories of nursing and models of nursing practice had been appearing in the literature, but most of the writings on these subjects were not available until the mid-seventies. Therefore, a search of the literature in the early seventies, when the groundwork for this curriculum was laid, did not provide answers to the numerous questions that were raised. Faculty struggled with concerns such as these: What is a conceptual framework and why do we need it? How is it developed? How can such a framework be used to organize nursing content, to develop courses, to select clinical learning experiences?

Then there were questions concerning process. How can thirty-five faculty members reach a consensus about essential concepts and essential clinical learnings? What are the first steps in preparing for change? How can individuals prepared as specialists teach in a curriculum that has no traditional specialty courses? And ad infinitum.

Over a period of six years, a committed faculty learned to work together, to debate and reach consensus, to try, to fail, to try again and finally succeed. The answers to the questions that had been raised, and to many more, evolved gradually. A totally new curriculum with a unique conceptual framework was developed along with the tools and techniques for evaluating student achievement and the effectiveness of the program. By June, 1982, seven classes had completed the program; its graduates are practicing successfully. Faculty, although not complacent because there is still much to be accomplished, are committed to the crisis theory framework as a model for practice as well as for curriculum.

The primary purpose of this book is not to sell the crisis model, however, but to provide a concrete illustration of the process of developing a conceptual framework and utilizing it in each step of curriculum development. To achieve this purpose, the contributors, all of whom were intimately involved with some aspect of the curriculum project, have assembled the information here that they wish had been available to them in the early 1970s. In addition to achieving this primary goal, the book may also interest the reader in exploring crisis theory as a model for practice and research as well as for an educational program.

Chapters 1 and 2 provide the theoretical basis for the chapters that follow. The decision to present curriculum theory from an historical perspective was made for two reasons. The first is probably the renewed interest in "roots" that is now apparent in many fields. The second surfaced when this book was still in the brainstorming stage. When the need for incorporating curriculum theory was mentioned, some contributors asked, "What are these curriculum theories we supposedly used? We know about philosophy, objectives, sequence, and continuity, but is there more to it than that? Where did the notion of integration come from?" The more the author of the first chapter researched the literature, and the more she delved into curriculum theory, the further back in nursing history her inquiries took her. Chapter 1 is the culmination of this extensive research. We believe the reader will find it sets the stage for the chapters that follow and adds meaning to the activities that are described.

The newest and probably the most difficult step in the curriculum development process is the formulation of the conceptual framework. Therefore, all of Chapter 2 is devoted to the ideas behind conceptual frameworks. The author is one of the leading authorities on the subject.

Chapters 3 through 9 are primarily a case study of the University of Connecticut experience. They describe faculty activities during each step in the process, giving examples of methods that were effective and those that failed, citing issues and problems that were resolved and those that continue to be debated. The pattern of chapters follows the model depicted in Figure 1.1, beginning with the formulation of a philosophy and the search for a conceptual framework, progressing to the translation of the framework into fully-developed courses, complete with objectives, content, learning experiences, and evaluative tools. Chapter 9 addresses the evaluation plan. Although the crisis model was originally developed for the undergraduate program, it was later adopted by the graduate program and provided an articulation between the two programs—this articulation is described in Chapter 10.

The crucial test of a framework for a nursing curriculum is the usefulness of that framework in nursing practice and research. Too often, a school's conceptual framework is described beautifully on paper but bears little relationship to student (or graduate) practice. If professional nursing practice based on a validated nursing model is to become a reality, baccalaureate curricula must be structured toward that end and be evaluated from that perspective. Therefore, Chapters 11, 12, and 13 have been included to illustrate the final steps in evaluating a curriculum design. Chapter 11 demonstrates the usefulness of the model in practice and research. Chapter

12 evaluates the model using the criteria presented in Chapter 2. Finally, Chapter 13, written by a University of Connecticut senior, provides the final test. It demonstrates the translation of the curriculum model into student practice.

The reader will notice that the terms "integrated curriculum" and "integrated approach" appear in a variety of places throughout the book. Integrated was a popular word in the seventies, and it was applied rather loosely to a variety of curriculum designs, including the University of Connecticut's. The so-called integrated curriculum of the seventies was one in which the various medical specialties were woven into each course rather than being separated into individual courses. The University of Connecticut curriculum goes beyond that; it has evolved from a unique nursing model unrelated to the traditional medical model. Therefore, "integrated" is a misnomer. Since this book, however, describes the curriculum process and problems as they were perceived at the time they were experienced and the term "integrated" was used freely by faculty at that time, it has not been deleted from this book.

There are instructional materials mentioned throughout the text; some of these may be available from the University of Connecticut School of Nursing, Storrs, Connecticut 06268.

Marguerite B. White

Acknowledgments

The writers wish to acknowledge the contributions of the many University of Connecticut faculty members, past and present, who generated ideas and participated in the development of the curriculum design and materials included within these pages. It would be impossible to give credit to some, individually, without slighting others who are equally deserving. We hope all who shared in this curriculum endeavor will derive satisfaction from reading this account of the experience and seeing a little bit of themselves in print.

Figures 3-1, 4-2, 6-1, 6-2, 6-3, 7-1, 7-2, 7-3, and 7-4 and Table 9-1 were compiled from materials developed by the University of Connecticut School of Nursing Faculty and appear with the permission of the University of Connecticut School of Nursing.

The curriculum project described in this book was funded by the Division of Nursing, Department of Health, Education, and Welfare (Nursing Special Project Grant No. D10-NU-00704).

Contributors

DOROTHY COBURN has a B.S. and M.S. from Boston University and is an assistant professor at the University of Connecticut. She has been on the University of Connecticut faculty since the beginning of the curriculum revision and was on the curriculum project staff for three years. She was team leader of the psychiatric nursing course in the former curriculum.

JACQUELINE FAWCETT received a B.S. from Boston University and an A.M. and Ph.D. from New York University. She is a Fellow of the American Academy of Nursing. As instructor and assistant professor at the University of Connecticut, she taught in both undergraduate and graduate programs. She is presently Associate Professor and Chairperson, Science and Role Development, University of Pennsylvania School of Nursing. Dr. Fawcett is the author of several publications dealing with conceptual models and theories of nursing.

EVELYN R. HAYES has a B.S. from Cornell University, an M.P.H. from the University of North Carolina School of Public Health, and a Ph.D. from Boston College. She is an associate professor at the University of Connecticut and teaches in both graduate and undergraduate programs. Dr. Hayes was senior level coordinator for two years. She is currently an NLN accreditation site visitor.

EDNA JOHNSON has a B.S. from the University of Minnesota and an M.S. from the University of North Caroline School of Public Health. She is an assistant professor at the University of Connecticut and is a certified Family Nurse Practitioner. She has had varied experiences in both service and education.

PAULINE HEBERT received bachelor's and master's degrees in nursing from the University of Connecticut and is currently a doctoral candidate in Instructional Media in the University of Connecticut School of Education. Miss Hebert was an independent practitioner for one year before joining the University of Connecticut faculty as instructor in charge of the simulated laboratory. She is currently employed by the Providence, Rhode Island Veterans Administration Hospital in the inservice education department.

JANE MURDOCK received a B.S. from the University of Utah and an M.S. from Boston University. She is currently a doctoral candidate at the University of Massachusetts School of Education, Center for Curriculum Studies, and is an assistant professor and Assistant Dean at the University of Connecticut School of Nursing. Mrs. Murdock was on the University of Massachusetts faculty before coming to the University of Connecticut. She was a member of the Curriculum Project Staff for three years and served for three years as the first senior level coordinator.

EILEEN MURPHY received a B.S. from Syracuse University, an M.S. from Boston University, and is currently a doctoral candidate in the Doctor of Nursing Science Program at Boston University. She is assistant professor and chairperson of the junior level at the University of Connecticut. Miss Murphy has been on the University of Connecticut faculty since the beginning of the curriculum project and was a member of the Curriculum Project Staff for three years.

PAMELA STACY is a 1981 graduate of the University of Connecticut School of Nursing. The paper from which chapter 13 of this book was adapted was an Independent Study project to fulfill one requirement for the Degree with Distinction Program.

LINDA R. SUESS received a B.S. from the University of Connecticut, an M.S. from the University of California at San Francisco, and is a doctoral student at Boston College. She is an assistant professor at the University of Connecticut and served for three years as the first junior level coordinator. She has also taught at the University of Vermont.

JANICE A. THIBODEAU received a B.S. degree from the University of Connecticut and an M.S. in medical/surgical psychiatric nursing from Boston University. She received an Ed.D. from the University of Massachusetts in the area of adult and higher education.

She is an ANA certified adult nurse practitioner and an associate
professor at the University of Connecticut where she is director of
the primary care practitioner program. Dr. Thibodeau has taught in
both undergraduate and graduate programs at the University of Connecticut. She was also an independent practitioner for a year. In
1977 she established a wellness center for Mansfield, Connecticut
senior citizens, which continues to operate successfully. She is an
NLN accredited site visitor.

1

Curriculum Development in Nursing: Historical Perspective

Jane Murdock

"The nurse or teacher who knows only of her own time and surroundings is not only deprived of an unfailing source of interest,
she may be unable to estimate and judge correctly the current
events whose tendency is likely to affect her own career. We
must know how our work of nursing arose; what lines it has followed and under what direction it has developed best. Possessing
this knowledge, each one may help to guide and influence its future on the highest lines, and in harmony with its historical mis-
sion" (Dock, 1920, p. 2).

Nursing faculty who participate in curriculum development are usually so absorbed in what they are doing at the moment that they give
little thought to the past. Yet, the resolution of current curriculum
problems is often enriched by exploring such questions as "How did
we begin to do this anyway?" "What got us started?" "Why did we
think it was necessary and important?" "Are the conditions the same
now as then?" (Seguel, 1966). Although answers to such historical
questions do not provide a complete picture of the curriculum development process, they do reveal whether we are still doing what we set
out to do and give us a broader perspective on the problems within our
contemporary context.

This chapter attempts to provide such a perspective in nursing
education by examining several distinct stages in the evolution of
nursing curricula in this country. After a brief overview of the

1

circumstances leading to the development of the early schools, each of these evolutionary stages will be analyzed in terms of their relationship to the growth of nursing as a discipline and to the progression of educational trends within the society at large.

THE DEVELOPMENT OF SCHOOLS OF NURSING IN THE UNITED STATES

During nursing's early history, there were no formal nursing schools. At first the family, and then various religious, military, and vocational groups shared the responsibility for inducting young nurses into the accumulated lore of nursing practice. In some instances, an organized program of training was provided, but the learners were apprentices—part employee, part pupil—rather than students (Stewart, 1943). When, in the latter part of the nineteenth century, it became apparent, that this apprenticeship system of education could no longer keep pace with the increasing demands of a complex industrial society, nursing schools began to emerge. The first school was founded by Florence Nightingale in England in 1860.

Shortly thereafter, the convergence of at least two societal factors provided the appropriate climate for the development of nursing schools in this country. The first was that conditions in city hospitals were deplorable. Nursing care was frequently left in the hands of drunken indigents or ex-convicts (Dolan, 1978). Dirt and squalor were the norm, and untimely death was often the outcome for those unfortunate enough to be hospitalized. The conditions within these institutions became prime targets for the reform-minded.

The second factor was the incipient emancipation of the Victorian woman. Many women sought meaningful work as volunteers in the reform movements which occurred both during and after the Civil War, while others were seeking to enter the work force in legitimate occupations (Dolan, 1978; Strauss, 1966). Teaching was one socially acceptable option open to these women; nursing and social work provided additional outlets.

Although in 1869 the American Medical Association discussed a recommendation to establish a training school for nurses in every hospital, and some physicians actually opened schools as early as 1872 (Dolan, 1978), it was not until 1873 that the first Nightingale schools appeared in this country. These schools were at Bellevue Hospital in New York City, New Haven State Hospital in New Haven, Connecticut, and Massachusetts General Hospital in Boston, Massachusetts (Kalisch & Kalisch, 1978).

In keeping with the Nightingale tradition, the schools were independent of the hospital, were governed by a lay board, and were usually administered by a woman who was both superintendent of the training school and chief nurse at the hospital. There was from the outset, however, some question of whether the primary aim of the schools was to provide charitable service for the improvement of hospitals or to offer a program for nursing education. Certainly, both motives were intricately intertwined. Effecting an appropriate balance between these two sometimes conflicting aims created many problems for nursing throughout its early developmental history.

FIRST STAGE IN CURRICULUM DEVELOPMENT: PIONEERING (1873–1893)

Stewart (1943) notes that the training programs in the early schools were based on a simple job analysis of nursing as it then existed and were aimed at assisting the student "to comprehend all that the nurse is required to know and do at the bedside of the sick" (p. 62). A list of the bedside functions to be mastered was distributed to the students and provided the focus for the content of the program of study. The list was copied from one used earlier by the Nightingale school in England.

Other than this list of the skills that all students were expected to master, there was little uniformity in the program of study within any one school, or between the several schools. The students were usually plunged headlong into the on-going activities of the ward, each one "taking her full share of the day's work and learning chiefly by trial and error" (Stewart, 1943, p. 105). Most of the instruction was conducted through these ward experiences, and little attention was paid either to their sequence or the relative proportion of each of the experiences within the total curriculum. The limited classroom instruction consisted of lectures by physicians and note taking. Recitations were conducted by the ward nursing staff (Stewart, 1943).

When seen from a contemporary viewpoint, these early schools and their curricula seem very primitive. However, they must be viewed within the context of the general educational milieu of the period. First, it should be noted that both the normal schools, established for the training of teachers, and the proprietary medical schools of the period had created a precedent for the development of single-purpose institutions to prepare for professional practice. The normal schools, in particular, were often held up as models for nursing to emulate (Dolan, 1978). Although professional schools were becoming more common, an apprenticeship system that did not rely on formal education was still considered an acceptable preparation for entry to practice in both medicine and law. Nursing's development in a modified apprenticeship format within the structure of a single-purpose school, then, was consistent with the prevailing approaches to professional education.

Second, neither pedagogy nor curriculum had as yet emerged as specialized fields of study. The prevailing approach to instruction relied upon the assumptions inherent within the classical tradition. Education was seen as a process of disciplining or strengthening the faculties of the mind through exercise, just as muscles are developed through use (Bode, 1940). In the context of this belief system, learning was thought to be largely a matter of memorizing words and reciting them back (Seguel, 1966). The variability of the nursing curricula or the rigidity of its methods of instruction were by no means noteworthy, for, in both, nursing education was in step with the standard educational practices of the time.

By 1893, however, concern over the declining quality of these educational programs had generated considerable uneasiness among nursing leaders. During the intervening decades, the number of schools had increased rapidly with a concomitant decrease in admission standards. In addition, economic realities had forced the schools to surrender operational control to their respective hospital boards. As a result of this new pattern of control, education had become a secondary, rather than a primary concern. Stewart (1943) observes, "In some cases . . . what was left was not even a good form of apprentice training" (p. 117). Although the program had been extended to two years in most of the schools, the theory portion still accounted for only two percent of the total required hours. The other 98 percent was devoted to scrubbing, cooking, and administering nursing care on the hospital wards (Kalisch & Kalisch, 1978).

The need for reform became essential, and the opportunity presented itself at the meeting of the International Congress of Charities, Correction, and Philanthropy held in association with the Chicago World's Fair of 1893. At this meeting, nursing leaders met together to discuss the status of nursing education. The papers presented on nursing at the Congress discussed the lack of uniformity in the curricula of the educational programs, the exploitation of students to meet the service needs of the hospitals, and the general lack of educational standards to sustain the quality of the schools. By the close of the Congress, forty superintendents of training schools had agreed to form an organization aimed at establishing and maintaining a universal standard of training (Stewart, 1943). The organization, called the American Society of Superintendents of Training Schools for Nurses (hereafter referred to as the Society of Superintendents or the Society), held its first convention the following year. The formation of this organization (an early ancestor of the National League for Nursing), and the development in 1896 of the Nurses' Associated Alumnae of the United States and Canada (the forerunner of the American Nurses' Association), marked the beginning of the era of standardization in nursing education.

SECOND STAGE IN CURRICULUM DEVELOPMENT: STANDARDIZATION (1893-1950)

The Early Period (1893-1917)

The early efforts of the nursing organizations were directed toward three fronts. First, The Associated Alumnae started a campaign to secure registration laws in each of the states. Once enacted, these were a strong force in regulating some of the conditions in the nursing schools. Because of these laws, for example, some schools raised their entrance requirements, broadened and strengthened their curricula, enlarged their clinical facilities, and improved their teaching. In addition, the state examinations, incorporated as part of the registration process, provided an incentive to students to do better work (Stewart, 1943).

Second, acting on a suggestion made during the Chicago Congress, and in the belief that the better educational preparation of those in charge of nursing schools would improve the quality of the educational offerings, the Society of Superintendents worked successfully to establish a post-graduate course for nurses at Teacher's College, Columbia University. Finally, the effort of the Society of Superintendents was directed toward establishing an improved and more standard curriculum in the schools. In the twenty-year period from 1893 to 1912, the course of study was lengthened to three years, and the content of the curriculum was extended considerably. Stewart (1943) reports that "the miscellaneous assortment of lectures and classes found in the earlier announcements was generally replaced by a classified list of courses with an instructor or lecturer assigned to each and with some progression from year to year" (p. 157).

In 1914, the Education Committee of the Society of Superintendents (by then renamed the National League of Nursing Education and hereafter referred to as the League) began preparing a standard curriculum to serve as a guide for nursing schools and also to represent to the public an idea of what was considered an acceptable standard of nursing education. With the publication of the Standard Curriculum for Schools of Nursing in 1917 the League reached a new level of refinement in its efforts to establish an improved and more standard nursing curriculum across the country.

The Standard Curriculum for Schools of Nursing (1917)

The Standard Curriculum was divided into two major sections. The first section outlined specific guidelines for the physical facilities, financial resources, and administrative control of the schools. Specific qualifications for both students and faculty, guidelines for student life, and recommended methods of teaching were also detailed. The second section presented a carefully worked out curriculum plan complete with objectives, content, methods, resources, and operational schedules. This was supplemented by a similar plan of practical instruction which outlined the time and sequence of the recommended experiences.

The sub-section on teaching was particularly innovative and reflected the increased educational sophistication of the nursing leadership. At least two significant factors contributed to this marked shift in educational perspective. The first was that the postgraduate program at Teacher's College was by now well into its second decade of operation and had generated a cadre of better prepared nurse educators. To a large extent, those responsible for setting the educational direction for nursing during this period were graduates of the Teacher's College program.

Secondly, by virtue of their contact at Teacher's College with such prominent figures as Edward L. Thorndike, John Dewey, and Frank McMurry, the nursing leadership had been directly exposed to, and shaped by, the mainstream of progressive educational thought. Stewart (1943) notes that "those who studied under such leaders were at first overpowered by the impact of new ideas that ran counter to former teachings and traditions, but gradually these ideas began to take hold in nursing as in other branches of education" (p. 146). For example, Thorndike's research on animal learning had effectively refuted the precepts of faculty psychology and opened the way for other conceptions of the learning process (Bode, 1940). Among these, Dewey's scientific orientation predominated. For Dewey the development of the ability to think was central to the educational process; acquiring knowledge was always secondary to the act of inquiry (Dewey, 1916).

Frank McMurry's impact on education lay in a somewhat different direction. Although he also denied the validity of faculty psychology, his approach to education was primarily rooted in the philosophy of Johann Herbart. As a Herbartian, McMurry believed that the mind actively creates a unity out of the raw materials of ideas presented to it. This belief led McMurry and other Herbartians to develop methods of instruction and techniques of curriculum development that would support the assimilation of knowledge and foster the correlation of the subject matter of the curriculum (Seguel, 1966). The Standard Curriculum reflected the influence of these prominent educators.

Although actual practices in the schools did not always measure up to the theoretical positions outlined, the Standard Curriculum did have a significant impact upon school improvement. Stewart (1943) reports that "results were evident not only in richer and better balanced curriculum content but in greater uniformity" (p. 223). Within a few years, however, circumstances within the schools, the profession, and the society at large indicated a need for revision of the curriculum.

Nursing education was brought to the critical attention of the public as a result of the participation of nurses on the front during World War I, and at home in the public health movement both during and after the war. These experiences accentuated the deficiencies in the existing educational system for preparing nurses. As a result, in 1919, a committee composed of leaders from nursing, public health, education, and hospital administration was funded by the Rockefeller Foundation to conduct a national study of nursing education. The report of this committee, published in 1923, and referred to as the Goldmark Report in honor of its director, Josephine Goldmark, made recommendations for changes in the education of public health nurses, and for nursing education in general (Goldmark, 1923). A number of these recommendations influenced the revision of the Standard Curriculum published by the League in 1927 (Stewart, 1943).

Other educational advances made between 1917 and 1927 had an additional impact upon this work. During this period, the study of curriculum had come into existence as a specialized field of study within educational theory. Educational historians (Caswell, 1966; Kliebard, 1968) credit Bobbitt (1918, 1924) and Charters (1923) with initiating systematic work in this field. Reflecting the more general movement toward efficiency underway in the society at large, and incorporating methods adapted from industry, these men formulated a new approach to curriculum development.

In contrast to those who preceded them, Bobbitt and Charters focused on the process of curriculum development rather than on the specific content or structure of the curriculum. Bobbitt took the lead in establishing this direction. Seguel (1966) observes:

> Using industry as his controlling metaphor, Bobbitt began to think about the curriculum. If (he theorized) the schools were a factory, the child the raw material, the ideal adult the finished product, the teacher an operative, the supervisor a foreman, and the superintendent a manager, then the curriculum could be thought of as whatever processing the raw material (the child) needed to change him into the finished product (the desired adult) (p. 80).

The key to Bobbitt's theory was this emphasis on a standard product, the ideal adult. He contended that the criteria for this ideal adult should be set by the community and could be determined by an analysis of adult activities (Seguel, 1966).

Following Bobbitt's general lead, Charters (1923) devoted a major portion of his professional career to developing and testing a specific method of curriculum construction. He recommended that teachers actively participate in the curriculum development process through an organized committee structure, and that they adopt the following methodology: determine the ideals and activities that constitute the major objectives; analyze and rank them in order of importance; determine the number that can be mastered in the time allotted; "collect the best practices of the race in teaching these ideals and activities"; and arrange materials in appropriate instructional order. This was the beginning of a sequential process for curriculum development. The approach served as a guide for the revision of the nursing curriculum, and generated an interest in curriculum theory which continues in nursing to the present day.

Curriculum for Schools of Nursing (1927)

In preparing for the work of revision, the League's Education Committee conducted an activity analysis in nursing and outlined in some detail the functions and qualifications expected of the rank and file nurse (Stewart, 1943). These constituted the practical objectives of the curriculum and served as the basis for reconstructing the course of study. Twenty-two subcommittees composed of nurses representing all parts of the country and all branches of the profession participated in the task of revision. Reports of these committees were published in The American Journal of Nursing, and reprints of the different outlines were made available so that nurses across the country were able to try out and to criticize the new courses before they were compiled in book form (National League of Nursing Education, 1927).

While the curriculum did not change dramatically, there were a number of shifts in emphasis which should be noted. First, the word "standard" was dropped from the title of the revision to reflect more accurately the intent of the publication; the League wished to make it clear that the publication was to be used as a guide—it was not a hard and fast requirement or a law as some had supposed to be true of the first edition (Stewart, 1943).

Second, as a result of the influence of the Goldmark report (1923), the idea of a basic course of studies common to all students was accepted as an operating norm. The elective specialties included as part of the final year of the program in the earlier edition were eliminated in the revision. It was recommended instead that the elements of these specialty areas, especially public health nursing, be included for all students (Stewart, 1943). Third, the hours of formal instruction were increased by about forty percent, and the ratio of the hours of theory and practice was changed from about 1 to 10, to 1 to 7 (Stewart, 1943).

A Curriculum Guide for Schools of Nursing (1937)

At the same time that this revision of the curriculum was being prepared, another effort toward reform was underway. With the Goldmark report (1923) as an impetus, and the Flexner report (1910) in medical education as a successful example of what could be done, the League sought a way to evaluate and grade schools of nursing across the country. The Committee on the Grading of Nursing Schools was established in 1926. The Committee, made up of representatives from nursing, medicine, education, and the lay public, had a task even wider than its name implied. As the diverse interests of the members were brought together, the Committee agreed to focus its study on the "ways and means for insuring an ample supply of nursing service of whatever type and quality is needed for adequate care of the patient, at a price within his reach" (Committee on the Grading of Nursing Schools, 1934, p. 16). Three major projects were conducted: a study of nursing economics, two gradings of nursing schools, and an activity analysis for nursing.

The findings of the Committee, published in 1934, documented an oversupply of nurses, inadequate wages, poor training, and a paucity of clinical resources for existing educational programs. They recommended (1) the reduction of the nurse supply and improvement of the quality of training; (2) replacement of students with graduates for routine ward duty; (3) assistance to hospitals to help meet costs of graduate services; and (4) public support for nursing education (Kalisch & Kalisch, 1978). Although the actual gradings were reported to the individual schools, the lists were not made public as the Flexner report had been. Instead, the Committee recommended that the League undertake the task of developing an accreditation program. Because of the widespread financial problems created by the depression, this project had to be postponed for several years (Stewart, 1943).

The next logical steps (Taylor, 1935) seemed to be a detailed study of what should be included in the education of nurses and the revision of the Curriculum. The theoretical guidelines to be employed in this reconstruction were published in The American Journal of Nursing (Smith, 1935). In contrast to the more mechanistic methods utilized in developing the 1927 revision, these guidelines reflected a new emphasis on philosophical exploration. Although the attitude of critical self-appraisal generated by the Goldmark (1923) and Grading Committee (1934) reports probably played a part in creating this more philosophical stance, it can perhaps be more directly attributed to changing perceptions among the curriculum theorists of the period. Smith (1935) observes:

> Curriculum workers . . . learned to rely upon the work of kinds of truth-seekers—the philosopher and the research worker . . . . The philosopher contributes a body of principles . . . . The researcher develops a body of technics helpful in meeting those recurring problems that are commonly found in most curriculum situations. The curriculum worker . . . cannot travel far without help from both (p. 461).

The effort to combine philosophy and technique was nowhere more evident than in the work of Hollis Caswell. Caswell (1935) described a method in which clearly identified aims were used to guide program development and foster consistency among the various elements of the curriculum. He asserted that curriculum development was essentially a matter of judgment rather than technique (Seguel, 1966). In the belief that these judgments would be enhanced by the widest possible participation in the decision-making process, he recommended that teachers and representatives of other interested professional and lay groups be actively involved (Caswell & Campbell, 1935). Caswell's methodology served as a guide for constructing the revision of the nursing curriculum initiated in 1934 and published in 1937 under the title A Curriculum Guide for Schools of Nursing.

A variety of committees and subcommittees carried out the 1937 revision under the direction of a central curriculum committee. About two hundred nurses as well as fifty or more doctors, librarians, dieticians, social workers, and representatives of other professional groups actively participated in the project. Stewart (1943) reports that "in addition, . . . over 700 study groups, with about 300 members in all, shared in the discussion and criticism of general bulletins and course outlines" (pp. 156–257). A series of articles published in The American Journal of Nursing also kept nurses around the country in touch with the work as it progressed.

One committee was assigned the difficult task of articulating a philosophy of education for nursing and condensing this into a statement of aims and objectives for the curriculum. The concept of adjustment was accepted as the overall aim of nursing education. As defined by the committee, the concept was active, positive, and involved changes in both the individual and his environment. It incorporated such progressive aims as the "releasing of capacity," the stimulation of growth and self-expression, participation in social life, the progressive reconstruction of experience and the "remaking of life," preparation for the duties and responsibilities of life, the enrichment of life experiences, and the promotion of individual happiness as well as social usefulness (Stewart, 1935, p. 273).

With the selection of the concept of adjustment as its guiding framework, nursing moved away from its traditional aims of discipline, service, practical utility, and technical efficiency, and closer to the democratic ideals expressed by the progressive educators of the period. Within this framework, other curriculum committees used a number of data sources (activity analysis, lists of traits and diseases, surveys of educational trends and practices) to develop specific curriculum objectives, specify standards for curriculum implementation, design an overall pattern of curriculum organization, and construct the individual courses of the program of study. While the overall organization of the program remained essentially the same, the substance of the courses did change considerably to keep pace with the advance of knowledge and changes in nursing practice.

Although the Curriculum Guide (1937) was well received and had an impact on school improvement, it was the last of its type to be published. A number of trends which had been developing since the turn of the century began to gain momentum in the 40s and 50s, causing the League to change its approach to the problems of nursing education. The first of these emerging trends to influence the curriculum was the development of collegiate schools of nursing.

Collegiate-based Schools

The first university-affiliated school of nursing was founded at the University of Minnesota in 1909. In fact, this was just a hospital diploma school added onto a university—no degree was offered until 1919 (Gray, 1960). It did, however, represent a turning of the educational tide. Following this, "the talk of 'better education' for nurses came, almost imperceptibly, to be transformed into pleas for 'university education'" (Davis et al., 1966, p. 146).

By 1920 at least 180 schools had some type of affiliation with higher education. In the majority of these, the affiliating institutions merely provided students from hospital schools with courses in the basic sciences and related areas. Some had arrangements whereby students could receive a degree upon completion of a hospital program and some additional college work. A few offered a combined academic and professional course, usually five years in length, leading to a bachelor of science degree (MacDonald, 1965).

Despite the efforts of a small, active, and vocal group of nursing educators to establish and maintain standards for the development of collegiate schools, only small gains were made during the 1930s and early 1940s. During the depression years, in particular, schools continued on a shoestring with much of their support coming from hospitals in payment for student services. Also, since there was a scarcity of prepared faculty, almost every collegiate program had to depend on hospital-based nursing personnel to teach and supervise students. As a result, the nursing faculty was greatly restricted in its development and control of the schools' curricula (MacDonald, 1965).

Although there were many problems, the movement toward university-based education gained increasing momentum during the 1940s. A prominent movement leader stated in 1943:

It seems probable that in nursing as in home economics, teaching, library work, and many other fields, a bachelor's degree will become in the near future a commonly accepted basic qualification for professional practice. There is no more reason to consider such a person a 'super-nurse' than to consider a young M.D. a 'super-doctor' (Stewart, 1943, p. 302).

Three major studies conducted after the Second World War (Brown, 1948; Committee on the Function of Nursing, 1948; Bridgman, 1953) recommended the expansion and improvement of collegiate education if nursing was to achieve an equal footing with other professions and fulfill its responsibilities in the health care system. These recommendations, in addition to an increased interest in nursing on the part of groups within higher education, lent support and contributed to the continuing advancement of collegiate nursing education during the following decades.

Accreditation

The Brown (1948) report recommended that "nursing make one of its first matters of important business the long overdue official examination of every school, that the lists of accredited schools be published and distributed as far as possible to every town and city of the United States. . . ." (p. 116). Nursing's movement toward accreditation as a means of quality control represented another emerging trend, one that would have a profound influence upon the future development of nursing curricula in the country.

Societal circumstances in 1948 were far more hospitable for accreditation than they had been previously. First, it had become increasingly clear that no one standard curriculum could satisfy the diversity of aims reflected in both diploma and collegiate education. (The problem would be compounded, of course, when associate degree programs were added to the picture in the 50s.) Second, since application of the curriculum guidelines was purely voluntary, there was no mechanism other than the State Board regulatory processes to evaluate compliance with the specified standards. A system of accreditation would provide a more effective means of sustaining the quality of nursing education. Finally, the resources for mounting a full-scale accreditation program were more readily available with the passing of the depression and war years.

In 1949, a joint board of six nursing organizations formed the Joint Committee on the Unification of Accreditation Activities. This group served as the impetus behind the development of the National Nursing Accrediting Service (Ozimek, 1974; Walsh, 1975). With the restructuring of the national organizations in 1952, the accrediting services were placed in the hands of the Division of Nursing Education of the newly-formed National League for Nursing (created by the merger of the National League of Nursing Education, the National Organization for Public Health Nursing, and the Association of Collegiate Schools of Nursing).

From its inception, accreditation was voluntary and was conducted in relation to criteria established by the profession. It featured self-study by the schools, on-site visitation for data collection, evaluation by a board of peers, and public disclosure of the outcome of the process through publication of lists of the accredited schools. Initially, a category called temporary accreditation was included in the listings. This was awarded for a five-year period on the assumption that, with assistance, many schools could improve their facilities and programs (Fagan, 1960). A School Improvement Program was launched to provide such assistance. As a result, more than one hundred schools upgraded themselves to full standard and more than five hundred were well along the way to that goal by the time the program was discontinued in 1957 (Sheahan, 1960).

A newly revised edition of the Curriculum Guide was due during this period. In 1950, however, the League made the concept of a standard curriculum obsolete by officially asserting that the faculty of each school, rather than the profession as a whole, should be responsible for curriculum development within the confines of standards established by the profession. This action inaugurated a new era in the evolution of nursing curricula in the country. Although the League's action had an impact on all types of nursing programs—diploma, associate degree, and baccalaureate—the remainder of this chapter will focus primarily on curriculum development in baccalaureate nursing education.

THIRD STAGE IN CURRICULUM DEVELOPMENT:
STRUCTURAL DIVERSITY (1950–1970)

Ongoing developments in education had a profound influence upon curriculum thought and practice in nursing during the 1950s and 60s.

For example, the group dynamics movement of the 1940s was instrumental in introducing a whole new approach to curriculum development. The focus shifted to the process of change rather than to the change itself and faculty became directly involved in that process (Conley, 1973). The League actively supported this new direction and provided a series of conferences to augment faculty skills in curriculum development. Published reports of the early conferences (Dept. of Services to Schools, National League of Nursing Education, 1950, 1951; Elliott, 1957) and of those conducted in more recent years (Dept. of Baccalaureate and Higher Degree Programs, National League for Nursing, 1974a; 1974b; 1974c; 1975a; 1975b; 1975c) have been widely used by the schools as a curriculum resource.

Another major influence that emerged during this time was the work of Ralph Tyler. His writings provided a link between past and present curricula in nursing history as well as in the curriculum field in general (Goodlad, 1968). He synthesized the ideas of such early curriculum scholars as Charters and Judd (with whom he worked) and developed the now-famous "Tyler rationale" for curriculum development. These ideas were refined and published in 1949 as a syllabus for a curriculum course he taught at the University of Chicago. This publication, Basic Principles of Curriculum and Instruction (1949), represented "a systematic resynthesis of progressive educational thought spanning earlier decades . . . [and] serves to this day as the definitive conceptual scheme for curriculum development" (Tanner & Tanner, 1975, p. 60).

The Tyler Rationale for Curriculum Development

Tyler's rationale provided the foundation for curriculum development in nursing and continues to do so to the present day. In Basic Principles of Curriculum and Instruction, Tyler posed four fundamental questions which must be answered in developing any curriculum and plan of instruction:

1. What educational purposes should the school seek to attain?
2. What educational experiences can be provided that are likely to attain these purposes?
3. How can these educational experiences be effectively organized?
4. How can we determine whether these purposes are being attained? (Tyler, 1949, p. 1)

He then goes on to outline methods for answering the questions. These methods, and not direct answers to the questions, constitute the Tyler rationale.

Tyler suggests that three major data sources—studies of learners studies of contemporary society, and recommendations from subject-matter specialists—be surveyed to elicit a comprehensive list of educational purposes. This list should then be filtered through two "screens"—a philosophy of education and a psychology of learning—to derive a realistic, noncontradictory list of achievable objectives for the program in question.

Tyler views these objectives as "general modes of reaction," rather than "specific habits to be acquired" (p. 43), and suggests that they be stated clearly "in terms which identify both the kind of behavior to be developed in the student and the content or area of life in which this behavior is to operate" (p. 48).

The selection of appropriate learning experiences is the next step. Tyler suggests a number of general principles:

1. The student must have experiences that give him an opportunity to practice the kind of behavior implied by the objective (p. 65).
2. The student must obtain satisfaction from carrying on the kind of behavior implied by the objectives (p. 66).
3. The reactions desired in the experience are within the range of possibility for the students involved (p. 67).
4. Many particular experiences can be used to attain the same educational objectives (p. 67).
5. The same learning experiences will usually bring about several outcomes (p. 67).

Once selected, these learning experiences must be organized in such a way that they reinforce each other. Tyler proposes three major criteria: continuity, sequence, and integration. Continuity refers to the "vertical reiteration of major curriculum elements" (p. 84). Sequence is related to continuity but is an extension of it; each experience builds upon preceding ones but goes "more broadly and deeply into the matters involved" (p. 85). Integration, "the horizontal relationship of curriculum experiences, . . . should . . . help the student increasingly to get a unified view and to unify his behavior in relation to the elements dealt with" (p. 85).

In working out the plan of organization it is necessary also to (1) identify the elements which serve as organizing threads of the curriculum (concepts, values, and skills); (2) identify the <u>organizing principles</u> by which these threads are to be woven together (continuity, sequence, integration, logical psychological order, increasing breadth of application, increasing range of activities, etc.); and (3) select the <u>main structural elements</u> in which the learning experiences are to be organized (subjects, broad fields or core curriculum designs in which the elements are organized in years, semesters, units, topics, and lessons).

Evaluation is also an important operation in curriculum development. Tyler's conception of evaluation has two important aspects: the appraisal of student behavior (p. 106), and the use of more than one method of appraisal; moreover, it is a "continuing cycle" (p. 123).

Tyler observes that the rationale can be used in developing an entire curriculum or any of its subparts. He recommends that it always involve the active participation of the faculty. In the concluding paragraph of the syllabus, he raises a commonly recurring question: "Must the sequence of steps followed be exactly as described in the syllabus?" His answer is an emphatic "No"

> The purpose of the rationale is to give a view of the elements that are involved in a program of instruction and their necessary interrelations. The program may be improved by attacks beginning at any point, providing the resulting modifications are followed through the related elements until eventually all aspects of the curriculum have been studied and appraised (p. 128).

The twenty-year period of the 50s and 60s was one of considerable experimentation and growth in the development of nursing curricula. There was widespread use of the Tyler rationale in these efforts. One notable example is the curriculum development project conducted at the University of Washington in the early 50s, under the direction of Ole Sand and Helen Belcher. Ralph Tyler provided direct consultation to this sophisticated application of his rationale. The reports of this study, published in three volumes (Sand, 1955; Tschudin, Belcher, & Nedelsky, 1958; Sand & Belcher, 1958), were a valuable resource for the faculty of other schools as they engaged in similar efforts.

In a guest editorial appearing in <u>Nursing Outlook</u> in 1957, Ole Sand observed that nurses were far more successful in their curriculum development efforts than their colleagues in other branches of higher education. In exploring the reasons for this success, he concluded:

The recency of nursing's advent in higher education is related to its leadership role. It has had no time to develop the complacency, slogans, or snobbishness that lead to a fossilized curriculum. A second reason for the excellence of nursing curriculum studies is that nursing has a much clearer notion about the ends it wants to achieve than most other groups have. One finds less energy expended upon the means as means. There is a willingness to study and to make choices of educational aims and to consider means as means to ends.

A third factor is the ability of nurse educators to interpret and appraise what they hear, see, read, and do about curriculum study in terms of a common rationale. One reason why so many university self-studies have gone nowhere is the lack of interest in and attention to the hard task of developing a common set of principles to guide curriculum study (p. 15).

Sand's latter point—that all nurses share a common set of principles to guide curriculum study—is a continuing strength and, even in the present day, sets nursing apart from other disciplines.

Curriculum Structure

Prior to 1950, most, if not all, nursing curricula had a similar organizational structure. Although curriculum content related to technical skills, environmental control, and a philosophy and code of ethics (Longway, 1972), the major focus was on disease and its control. The courses were structured either in relation to specific diseases (tuberculosis nursing), body-systems (orthopedic nursing), or patient care areas (pediatric nursing). Although this emphasis continued in many schools during the 50s and 60s, other structural forms also appeared. Stevens (1971) observes that they were essentially of four types: logistic, operational, problematic, and dialectical.

The logistic mode of curriculum organization is exemplified in the disease, body systems, or patient care area approaches. The curriculum is built upon the individual parts of the nurse's responsibility; from this it is hoped that the student will come to view the totality. In this mode the nurse, the student, and the patient are all subsidiary to the health-illness struggle.

In the operational mode the student becomes the center of attention. The curriculum is organized in relation to the student's perceived learning needs. The focus is not upon disease or the patient, but on the nurse's operations. Within this organizational scheme, patient cases, either real or simulated, often serve as centers for learning.

The third type of organization focuses on the problems rather than on the patient, the disease, or the student. This mode has its origins in the work of John Dewey (1916) and was stimulated in nursing at this time by the publication of Abdellah's (1960) conceptualization of "21 Nursing Problems"; both sources focus on the act of inquiry, or the problem-solving method, rather than content (Stevens, 1971).

In the final mode, the dialectical, the organizing principle is some synthesizing "whole" such as the developmental life span of man, or the health-illness continuum. Within this organizational pattern, the student gains a more and more comprehensive understanding of the patient as she progresses through the curriculum. Stevens (1979) observes that the aim of such a curriculum is "to teach the nurse to interact effectively with the whole person" (p. 153). The patient, therefore, becomes the central focus within this mode of curriculum organization.

The structural diversity of the nursing curricula of this period reflects the variability of the philosophy and psychology of learning of the faculties involved in their development. This level of diversity of outcome also demonstrates the effectiveness of the Tyler rationale as a "management system" (Huebner, 1976, p. 161) for balancing the tensions between objectives arising from three data sources—learners, society, and subject matter. Whereas the logistic mode gives preference to subject matter, and the operational mode puts the learner in the forefront, the problematic and dialectic modes make the problems of society, and of individuals within the society, the organizing focus of the curriculum. Within the framework of the Tyler rationale, individual faculties were able to make the choices most appropriate for their time and place. As nursing entered the 70s, the Tyler rationale continued to serve as a theoretical foundation for curriculum development. However, both the rationale and the curricula that have emerged from its use have undergone a number of evolutionary changes.

In the late 60s, stimulated by a sense of urgency to establish a theoretical foundation for nursing practice, and encouraged perhaps by the general interest in the conceptualization of all disciplines, a number of nurses began the work of building conceptual frameworks both to guide nursing practice and to integrate the nursing curriculum. Continuing efforts in this direction characterize the contemporary era.

FOURTH STAGE IN CURRICULUM DEVELOPMENT:
CONCEPTUALIZATION, INTEGRATION, AND NURSING MODELS
(1970–   )

Discussions of curriculum integration have appeared in the nursing literature for many years, for example, in the 1937 Curriculum Guide (p. 69). However, in practice, such attempts at integration did not usually break down the tight compartmentalization characteristic of the logistic mode.

Heidgerken observed in 1955 that a truly integrated program requires a "synthesis of content from the different areas of knowledge organized around some unifying principle" (p. 129). Most educators now agree that a conceptual framework provides that unifying principle; "today we have moved to the adoption of frameworks around which we endeavor to weave the whole cloth" (Styles, 1976, p. 739).

What was only a dream in 1955 has been a formal requirement for program accreditation since 1972. A new criterion, added for the first time in 1972, stated "the curriculum plan is based on a conceptual framework(s) consistent with the stated philosophy, purposes, and objectives of the program(s)" (National League for Nursing, 1972, p. 8). The most recent edition of the criteria (National League for Nursing, 1977) reiterates the intent: "The curriculum implements the philosophy, purposes, and objectives of the program and is developed within a conceptual framework" (p. 13).

Changes occurring in nursing education continue to reflect the general educational milieu. In 1959, Jerome Bruner chaired a national conference that explored ways of improving science education. A pervading theme that emerged from this conference was that curriculum reform should follow the "structure" of each discipline, as Bruner suggested (1960, p. 31). Two curriculum theorists of the period, Joseph Schwab (1962; 1964) and Philip Phenix (1964), concurred.

This quest for structure, in fact, represents a search for synthesis. These educational theorists reasoned that by understanding the fundamental and general ideas that constitute a discipline, the learner would be able to continually broaden and deepen his knowledge. Torres adopts the same view (1974, p. 6).

Although these external educational events had a profound influence on the direction of curriculum development in nursing, other internal events also had an impact. The 1960s and 1970s were decades of professional awakening in nursing, a time during which the critical analysis of nursing's professional status was a key concern.

During this period it became clear to many that if nursing was indeed to be considered a profession, nurses should be able to clearly identify and continually develop the theoretical body of knowledge upon which their practice rests. Many nurse scholars are now engaged in these theoretical explorations. Nursing models are being developed and validated to provide a base for professional nursing practice.

The dynamic interaction of these internal and external events has led to the intimate linking of the notions of conceptual structure, curriculum integration, and practice based on a nursing model. The scheme outlined in figure 1-1 accurately reflects contemporary nursing practices; it is based on, consistent with, but modified from Tyler's rationale of 1949.

Data Sources. The three sources outlined in the Tyler rationale—learners, society, and subject matter—provide the data for developing the philosophy, objectives, and conceptual framework of the curriculum.

Philosophy. Philosophy is now placed in a primary position in nursing's curriculum rationale, a view consistent with current curriculum thought. Goodlad & Richter (1966) have reexamined Tyler's work and present a revised conceptual system for dealing with problems of curriculum and instruction. They contend that, since values and philosophical positions inevitably enter into all steps in curriculum planning, these value positions should serve as "the primary data-source in selecting purposes for the school and as a data-source in making all subsequent curricular decisions" (p. 27). Thus, values are viewed as the base or foundation of the curriculum development process rather than a "screen" for objectives as in the Tyler rationale—more a change of emphasis than intent.

A philosophy, then, is the faculty's statement of those beliefs and values upon which the curriculum is based. It should be consistent with the philosophy of the parent institution and reflect value positions in relation to the nature of man, society, health, nursing, knowledge, learning, and teaching. When committed to writing, the statement of philosophy brings the faculty's value system to a conscious level. Dewey (1916) provided an apt definition when he described philosophy as "thinking which has become conscious of itself" (p. 381).

Objectives. The objectives of the curriculum are derived from the system of beliefs stated in the philosophy and spell out the

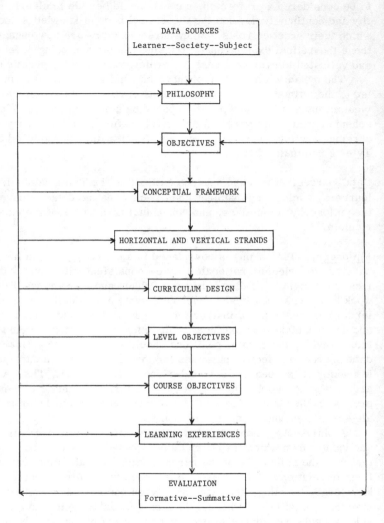

```
                    ┌─────────────────────────┐
                    │      DATA SOURCES       │
                    │ Learner--Society--Subject│
                    └─────────────────────────┘
                                 │
                                 ▼
                         ┌──────────────┐
          ┌──────────────│  PHILOSOPHY  │
          │              └──────────────┘
          │                     │
          │                     ▼
          │    ┌────────────────────────────────────┐
          │    │            OBJECTIVES              │◄───┐
          │    └────────────────────────────────────┘    │
          │                     │                         │
          │                     ▼                         │
          │      ┌──────────────────────────┐            │
          ├─────►│   CONCEPTUAL FRAMEWORK    │            │
          │      └──────────────────────────┘            │
          │                     │                         │
          │                     ▼                         │
          │   ┌───────────────────────────────────┐      │
          ├──►│ HORIZONTAL AND VERTICAL STRANDS   │      │
          │   └───────────────────────────────────┘      │
          │                     │                         │
          │                     ▼                         │
          │       ┌──────────────────────┐               │
          ├──────►│   CURRICULUM DESIGN   │               │
          │       └──────────────────────┘               │
          │                     │                         │
          │                     ▼                         │
          │        ┌────────────────────┐                │
          ├───────►│  LEVEL OBJECTIVES  │                │
          │        └────────────────────┘                │
          │                     │                         │
          │                     ▼                         │
          │        ┌────────────────────┐                │
          ├───────►│  COURSE OBJECTIVES │                │
          │        └────────────────────┘                │
          │                     │                         │
          │                     ▼                         │
          │     ┌────────────────────────┐               │
          ├────►│  LEARNING EXPERIENCES  │               │
          │     └────────────────────────┘               │
          │                     │                         │
          │                     ▼                         │
          │     ┌────────────────────────┐               │
          └────►│       EVALUATION       │◄──────────────┘
                │  Formative--Summative  │
                └────────────────────────┘
```

FIGURE 1-1. Nursing's rationale for curriculum development.

characteristics expected of the graduate. The overall program objectives are usually quite general. Increasing levels of specificity are achieved as these general objectives are translated into level, course, and unit objectives within the subelements of the program. The works of Bloom (1956), Krathwohl et al. (1964), Harrow (1972), Gronlund (1970), and Mager (1962) have been particularly useful in developing objectives that have behavior and content dimensions.

Conceptual Framework. The conceptual framework stems from the program's philosophy and, ideally, is a concise statement or diagram depicting the major concepts, skills, and values that the faculty defines as essential to nursing (Kelley, 1975). It is used to structure the courses of the curriculum and to provide a framework within which to view nursing practice.

The conceptual framework is probably the least well understood element within nursing's curriculum rationale. Consequently, the following chapter is devoted entirely to an elaboration of the use of conceptual frameworks both in nursing practice and nursing education. One general point should be made here however. Although the term conceptual framework is not specifically used in the Tyler rationale, Tyler's notion of "organizing elements" is somewhat analogous; both are elaborations of the essential concepts, skills, and values that provide structure to the curriculum. In each instance the terms are used to refer to a subelement of the curriculum development process.

However, other curriculum theorists, for example Hilda Taba (1962), use the term conceptual framework in an entirely different context. Rather than referring to a subelement of the curriculum development process, the term is used to describe the entire process. In this instance, a conceptual framework outlines the major elements involved in the overall process of curriculum development. Each use of the term is appropriate, but in order to avoid confusion it is important to distinguish between them.

Horizontal and Vertical Strands. Curriculum strands are highly synthesized constructs derived from the conceptual framework and used as organizing threads for the curriculum. Vertical strands provide for the progression of ideas in the curriculum and are related to Tyler's notions of continuity and sequence. Horizontal strands contain concepts which need to be used in most learning experiences and are related to Tyler's notion of integration. Whether a particular strand is considered horizontal or vertical is a matter of faculty choice. Careful identification of both vertical and horizontal strands brings coherence to the curriculum design and facilitates the development of level, course, and unit objectives.

Curriculum Design. The term "curriculum design" refers to the way in which different elements (for example, courses or units) of the curriculum are arranged in relation to one another. As Stevens (1971) demonstrated, different design options place varying degrees of emphasis on the learner, society, and subject matter. The choice of curriculum design is intimately linked to the program's philosophy, objectives, and conceptual framework. Some recent innovative designs allow for variable entry and exit points, permit different functional options, provide for continuous progress based on mastery, focus on problem solving and decision making, or emphasize the integration of knowledge.

Learning Experiences. Learning experiences can occur within the classroom and in a variety of practice settings. Regardless of the setting, however, all learning experiences should be planned to meet specific objectives, and should offer the student an opportunity to practice the behavior implied in the objective. The beliefs about learning held by the faculty will strongly influence the nature of the experiences planned.

Evaluation. Evaluation is an essential component of the curriculum process, providing feedback about the outcomes of the nursing program. Ideally, it is a continuous process and includes both formative and summative evaluation methods. Formative evaluation provides an appraisal of ongoing events and permits continuous feedback and improvement. Summative evaluation measures the extent to which the objectives of the program or some of its larger subunits have been achieved.

SUMMARY

This chapter has traced the evolution of the nursing curriculum from the time of the founding of the first schools in this country in 1873 until the present day. It has, in addition, related this evolutionary development to the progression of educational theory and the continuous growth of the nursing profession. It is hoped that this exploration of the past will assist in bringing nursing's present curriculum practices into sharper focus.

> To have a curriculum history . . . is not to fix names, dates, and events into our memories or merely to set them down in written form, it is to add one invaluable way of giving shape and meaning to the welter of activities that now fall into the category of curriculum activities (Kliebard, 1976, p. 248).

2

Why a Conceptual Framework?

Jacqueline Fawcett

This chapter deals with the general characteristics of conceptual frameworks, including a definition of the term, some distinctions between conceptual frameworks and philosophy and theory, and the functions of a conceptual framework. Emphasis is placed on the role of conceptual frameworks in curriculum design. In addition, a plan for the analysis and evaluation of conceptual frameworks of nursing is presented.

DEFINITION OF CONCEPTUAL FRAMEWORK

The term conceptual framework, and synonymous terms such as conceptual model, conceptual system, or conceptual scheme, refer to global ideas about individuals, groups, situations, and events of interest to a science. These phenomena are classified into concepts, which can be defined as words that bring forth mental images of the properties of things. Concepts are then linked to form propositions that state their interrelationships. These statements constitute the

---

Portions of this chapter were taken from Fawcett, J. A framework for analysis and evaluation of conceptual models of nursing. Nurse Educator, 5(6), 10-14, Nov.-Dec. 1980. © Jacqueline Fawcett.

basic assumptions of a science. A conceptual framework may, therefore, be defined as a set of concepts and the assumptions that integrate them into a meaningful configuration (Nye & Berardo, 1966, p. 3).

The concepts of a conceptual framework are highly abstract and usually are not directly observable in the real world. Similarly, the assumptions linking the concepts are abstract generalizations that are not immediately testable. By identifying and describing relevant phenomena, a conceptual framework provides a perspective for scientists, telling them what to look at and speculate about. It is a view of how phenomena are put together and how they work. Each conceptual framework alters how the world is viewed and what aspects of the world are of interest (Redman, 1974; Rogers, 1973). It is not unusual to find that more than one discipline or school of thought is interested in the same concepts. What distinguishes these fields of inquiry are different definitions and different measures of the concepts, as well as different assumptions linking the concepts.

Conceptual frameworks often evolve from inductive insights about phenomena of interest to a scientist. Reilly (1975) claimed that they were primarily derived from empirical data and intuition, often initially within the frame of reference of a related discipline. The synthesis that occurs in the development of a new conceptual framework, however, results in a product unique to the field. Deduction may also play a part in the continuing developing of a conceptual framework, especially as concepts and their connecting statements are clarified and refined.

While the specific functions of conceptual frameworks will be discussed later in this chapter, it is worth emphasizing here that they are useful to scientists. Their usefulness comes from the organization they provide for the knowledge of a field of inquiry. The global concepts of a framework may be thought of as outline headings for additional information gathered from theoretical formulations (the speculation, theories, and laws that make up the subject matter of a discipline) and empirical observations. Conceptual frameworks are also useful as general guides for scientists' activities, since the concepts and their connections provide a particular view of things. This guides scientists' observations and helps them interpret what they see. This also gives direction to the search for solutions to problems and provides general criteria for knowing when and how effectively a problem is solved.

The Conceptual Frameworks of Nursing

Peterson (1977) and Hall (1979) link the development of conceptual frameworks of nursing with interest in conceptualizing nursing as a distinct discipline and the concomitant introduction of ideas about nursing theory. They note that the widespread interest in conceptual frameworks is a reflection of the National League for Nursing's requirement for accreditation that curricula be based on conceptual frameworks. Thus, conceptual frameworks of nursing have evolved as an attempt to identify and describe the domain of nursing knowledge, which recently was characterized as study of "the wholeness or health of humans, recognizing that humans are in continuous interaction with their environments" (Donaldson & Crowley, 1978, p. 119). Within this domain, four essential concepts have been identified (Yura & Torres, 1975) as the specific phenomena of interest to nursing science: person, environment, health, and nursing. (For Yura and Torres's terms "man" and "society," the terms "person" and "environment" have been substituted here to avoid the use of the sexist term "man" and to express more fully the ideas inherent in the term "society.")

Each conceptual framework of nursing strives to define and describe "person" and "environment" as well as their interrelation. Every conceptual framework presents a definition of health, with some describing both the well and the ill person and environments conducive or detrimental to health. Each also identifies a set of specific goals of nursing, which are frequently derived from the definition of health presented by the framework. Finally, each conceptual framework spells out its version of the nursing process, often in considerable detail.

The works of several nurse scholars are currently recognized as conceptual frameworks. Among the best known are Johnson's Behavioral Systems Model (Johnson, 1980), King's (1981) Social Systems Model, Orem's (1980) Self-Care Model, Rogers' (1970) Life Process Model, and Roy's (1976) Adaptation Model. Other conceptual frameworks have been presented and reviewed in books by The Nursing Development Conference Group (1979), The Nursing Theories Conference Group (1980), Riehl and Roy (1980), and Stevens (1979). Each of these frameworks represents a different school of thought. As such, it is not surprising that each operationalizes the four essential concepts differently and links these concepts with diverse assumptions. In addition to these widely known conceptual frameworks, many schools of nursing are developing independent frameworks derived from the particular philosophical beliefs of their faculties (Hall, 1979).

DISTINCTIONS BETWEEN CONCEPTUAL FRAMEWORK AND PHILOSOPHY

A conceptual framework is not a philosophy. Philosophies are concerned with such metaphysical issues as the purpose of life, the nature of being and of reality, and the limits of knowledge. They set forth the beliefs and assumptions underlying values by stating "shoulds" and "oughts" about these issues. A philosophy is derived from personal experience and the contemplative comparisons of one's experiences with those of others (Chater, 1975; Silva, 1977).

A philosophy is not only different from a conceptual framework, it is not even part of one. Indeed, as Chater (1975, p. 429) pointed out, "values per se have no place within a conceptual framework." Rather, conceptual frameworks are derived from philosophies, and represent the translation of values into the identification and description of relevant concepts (McKay, 1975). Thus, the philosophical stance of a field of inquiry influences the structure and content of its body of knowledge by directing the explication of concepts and assumptions. Different philosophies lead to different conceptual frameworks.

Since philosophies are made up of metaphysical belief statements, they cannot be tested empirically. This means they cannot provide the validated knowledge that scientists need for their various activities. For a science is by definition composed of knowledge that is empirically testable. Similarly, the practice of a profession related to a science has as its base a body of scientific knowledge. Thus, while the philosophical stance of a field of inquiry influences the development of its knowledge, it does not comprise its scientific knowledge.

Philosophies of Nursing

A philosophy of nursing is a statement of beliefs and values about the metaphysical issues surrounding the essential concepts of nursing. Philosophies of nursing set forth beliefs and values about person, environment, health, and nursing. In the case of philosophies underlying nursing education, the statements extend to the purpose of professional education as well as to facilitation of teaching and learning (Torres & Yura, 1975). These philosophical statements are the first step in the development of nursing curricula. The philosophy of a school of nursing leads to identification of program purposes and characteristics of its graduates, as well as to the major ideas to be defined and described in the conceptual framework. However, philosophies of nursing do not represent the empirically tested knowledge needed for advancement of nursing science and for the practice of professional nursing.

DISTINCTIONS BETWEEN CONCEPTUAL FRAMEWORK AND THEORY

A conceptual framework is also not a theory. A theory is formally defined as "a set of interrelated constructs (concepts), definitions, and propositions that present a systematic view of phenomena by specifying relations among variables" (Kerlinger, 1973, p. 9). A theory postulates specific relationships among concepts and is a description, explanation, or prediction about the linkages among phenomena. In a practice discipline, theories may also be prescriptions that specify the activities necessary to achieve the goals of its practitioners (Dickoff & James, 1968). Moreover, according to Homans (1964), the propositions of a theory must form a deductive system which explains how change in the values of one concept are associated with change in the values of another concept.

Theories are derived from conceptual frameworks, just as the frameworks are derived from philosophies. The general, abstract, identification and descriptions of phenomena and their interrelationships provided by conceptual frameworks represent the first step in the development of the more concrete theoretical formulations needed for scientific activities.

The crucial distinction between a conceptual framework and a theory lies in its level of abstraction. A theory is a set of specific concrete concepts, along with their definitions and the propositions that link them. A theory also provides greater specification of phenomena and more detailed explanations of postulated relationships than a conceptual framework does. Furthermore, a conceptual framework is not testable. Its global concepts and their connections are too abstract for testing in the real world: only theories are specific enough to be testable. Even theories, however, may not be immediately testable, for empirical testing requires that concepts have measurable definitions and that the statements linking these variables be somehow observable. Therefore, only those theories that can generate hypotheses—theoretical statements containing operationally defined concepts and explicating observable relations—can be tested. Since only this kind of theory can be validated, it is the kind needed for a discipline having a practice component. For practice requires that theory be validated.

A conceptual framework embodies the world view, or paradigm, of a discipline or school of thought. Each theory derived from the framework—and there are usually several—explicates some or all of the paradigm's phenomena within a limited range. A theory is both more precise and more limited in scope than its parent framework. Although some people consider conceptual frameworks to be what Merton (1957) called "grand theories"—global orientations that attempt to explain a totality of events—the position adopted here is that conceptual frameworks are too abstract to be considered to be theories. As used here, the term "theory" refers to Merton's "theory of the middle range"—speculations concerned with relatively narrow ranges of data.

Nursing Theories

Nursing theories are most appropriately derived from the conceptual frameworks of nursing and may be defined as sets of interrelated propositions and definitions that present systematic views of the essential concepts of nursing—person, environment, health, nursing—by specifying relations among relevant variables (Fawcett, 1978a, p. 26). Currently, no unique nursing theories are evident. Given the present attention to theory construction in nursing, however, it is anticipated that nurse scholars will soon successfully establish a body of unique nursing knowledge.

Meanwhile, nursing must rely on theory borrowed from other disciplines like education, psychology, sociology, biology, physics, and chemistry. One problem with this strategy is that these theories have not generally been tested with the people and events found in nursing situations. Thus, it is not clear whether a theory that is valid in a different setting holds in nursing. A more serious problem is that theories borrowed from other disciplines deal with phenomena of interest to that subject. Thus, sociological theories deal with people's social interactions, while psychological theories deal with intrapsychic processes, and biological theories deal with physiological events. None of these disciplines claims interest in the "wholeness or health of humans" which Donaldson & Crowley (1978, p. 110) define as the domain of nursing. These borrowed theories force nurses to consider the person in a piecemeal fashion. Clearly, what is needed is a theory that deals with the person as a total being in continuous interaction with the surrounding environment.

FUNCTIONS OF A CONCEPTUAL FRAMEWORK

Conceptual frameworks are tools which allow us to comprehend something in its totality, as, for example, the whole universe or all of behavior. Since the human mind is finite, and since it is with the mind that we comprehend, conceptual frameworks help us to identify, as general guidelines only, those phenomena that are of importance at any particular time and in any particular situation (Rosenblueth & Wiener, 1945).

In nursing, conceptual frameworks are beginning to be used as general guides for the design and implementation of educational programs, research projects, clinical nursing practice, and administrative systems. The particular curriculum, research problem, practice situation, or management setting will dictate the explanations needed to fill in the outline provided by the framework. The conceptual frameworks of nursing are especially important at this time in the evolution of nursing science because they provide a distinct focus for nursing and so help to clarify the differences between nursing and other health professions.

Conceptual Frameworks and Nursing Education

A curriculum is a planned program of study in an academic discipline. Curricula are guided by implicit, if not explicit, philosophical statements of what is valued in the educational process. However, philosophies of educational programs cannot serve as the basis for such concrete curriculum decisions as course objectives, content, and sequence for, as was pointed out earlier, philosophies contain only metaphysical statements of values and beliefs—statements that are not testable.

Decisions about a curriculum usually flow from the body of knowledge of a discipline. In many fields of study, well-known theoretical formulations and methods of inquiry can be ordered hierarchically so that course content and sequence are easily determined. The emerging discipline of nursing has not been so fortunate. Ten years ago, Sr. Madeleine Clemence Vaillot (1970) noted, "the nurse educator faced with the immediate problem of developing a professional program in a new university has no well-established theories of nursing on which to base curriculum construction" (p. 235). Today, nurse educators are somewhat more fortunate in that they can choose one of the existing conceptual frameworks of nursing as the organizing plan for the curriculum. Indeed, two surveys (Hall, 1979; Riehl, 1980) revealed that many schools of nursing now use a recognized conceptual framework such as Rogers, Orem, King, Johnson, or Roy as the basis for the curriculum. Other schools responding to the questionnaire indicated they are developing their own frameworks, several of which are based on stress adaptation and systems ideas from other disciplines.

When used in nursing education, the primary purpose of a conceptual framework is to organize curriculum content and learning activities. Redman (1974) pointed out that nurse educators implicitly assume that current conceptual frameworks result in more efficient and effective achievement of nursing's goals than did previous curriculum patterns. In many schools, the validity of that assumption remains to be tested. In others, extensive evaluation programs have documented the effectiveness of curriculum plans based on conceptual frameworks.

The conceptual framework should be considered the sine qua non of curriculum construction. Generally, it can be used to plan the curriculum, to select instructional materials, and to guide student-teacher interaction (Bush, 1979). McKay (1975) pointed out more specific functions of conceptual frameworks in the educational process, stating "the framework defines the relationships among the factors involved in the program. It identifies priority concepts, indicates logical sequence for course progression, and implies the method of inquiry, the nature of the support required, and the format of the evaluation" (p. 31). In addition, the conceptual framework of a curriculum provides the structure for program objectives, course selection and content, learning activities, and teaching strategies (Roy, 1973). The framework also helps to identify the always elusive levels of nursing practice within one program, such as the junior and senior years of a baccalaureate program, as well as the distinctions among types of nursing programs, including associate degree, baccalaureate, master's, and doctoral programs (Reilly, 1975; Vaillot, 1970).

When a conceptual framework is used for curriculum construction, it must encompass general ideas about education and the teaching-learning process as well as content from the discipline of nursing (Bush, 1979; Wu, 1979). Thus, connections need to be made among the student, the setting, and the subject matter (Chater, 1975) as well as nursing's four essential concepts of person, environment, health and nursing. One way to accomplish this is to further delineate the essential concepts as they are described in the recognized conceptual frameworks of nursing. Person could then encompass the client, the student, and the educator. Environment would consider not only the client's surroundings, but also the settings for educational activities. The concept of health might be construed to mean the student's and the faculty member's health as well as the client's. Nursing could focus on the nursing process and on the teaching-learning process.

As each of the essential concepts is further specified, a list of progressively less abstract concepts evolves, providing the building blocks of the curriculum. The lower level concepts are then interrelated by various theoretical formulations. Thus, the concepts of the conceptual framework identify broad areas of content for the curriculum. For example, if the person were viewed as a biopsychosocial being, course content would include knowledge about the biology of humans, their psychological processes, and social relations. Less abstract concepts then specify the particular theories to be taught. For example, if the environment was seen as a source of stimuli to which the person must respond in certain ways in order for adaptation to occur, course content would be drawn from the behaviorist school of thought, with its focus on stimulus-response theories.

The concepts and their connecting statements also direct the sequence of courses. For example, if health was viewed as a continuum from peak wellness to acute illness each course could consider a different segment of the continuum. Moreover, if, for example, the faculty believed that effective learning proceeds along a line from simple to complex, conceptual framework concepts could then be selected as strands that encompass increasingly difficult content.

The most important function of the conceptual framework used for nursing education is that it "provides the student and thus the graduate with a framework for nursing practice" (Peterson, 1977, p. 29). This is noteworthy because, as pointed out earlier, conceptual frameworks of nursing can provide a uniquely nursing-oriented focus to the nurse's activities. One result of the use of conceptual frameworks, then, is an increase in nurses' confidence that what they are doing is nursing, and not medicine, or social work, or any other health profession.

The remaining chapters in this book will present a case study of the use of a conceptual framework developed by the faculty of the University of Connecticut School of Nursing. These chapters will illustrate how the conceptual framework guided the curriculum plan and will outline the various theoretical materials used to provide the concrete information needed for implementation of the curriculum. The grid depicting the concepts taught in each nursing course, illustrated in Figures 4-1 and 6-3, highlights the direction for course selection, content, and sequence provided by the conceptual framework.

Conceptual Frameworks and Research

Conceptual frameworks provide the basic conceptual, instrumental, and methodological rules for research in a discipline. Specifically, as Schlotfeldt (1975) outlined, the conceptual framework selected for any study influences:

> (1) the precise nature of the problem to be studied, or the purposes to be fulfilled by the investigation, or both; (2) the phenomena to be studied; (3) the research techniques to be employed and the research tools to be used; (4) the settings in which data are to be gathered and the subjects who are to provide the data; (5) the methods to be employed in reducing and analyzing the data; and (6) the nature of contributions that the research will make to the advancement of knowledge (p. 7).

In essence, the conceptual framework is the skeleton of the study. It identifies the concepts from which specific variables are derived for the investigation and also describes the assumptions that serve as the basis for the propositions from which testable hypotheses are deduced. The subject matter of a particular study might be one concept or the relations between two or more of nursing's essential concepts. Theoretical formulations from other disciplines may be tested in nursing situations or the focus of study might be construction and testing of a unique nursing theory.

The conceptual framework adopted by a school of nursing can provide structure for faculty and student research. When the research program of a school is based on one framework, much progress can be made in the building and testing of theories that describe, explain, and predict the phenomena of nursing science and prescribe the activities of its practitioners from the perspective of that school of thought.

Conceptual Frameworks and Clinical Practice

Conceptual frameworks of nursing also provide models of practice by identifying the goals of practice and the process to be followed in achieving those goals. Nursing care is the real world expression of the framework in all its ramifications. Broncatello (1980, p. 13) stated, "a conceptual model . . . elucidates possible relationships within the client situation upon which nursing diagnoses may be made and provides direction for nursing intervention." Thus, a conceptual framework guides all aspects of clinical practice from such basic skills as health assessment to the most advanced, sophisticated nursing interventions, as when caring for multiple problem families. The framework tells the clinician what to look at when interacting with clients, how to interpret observations, how to plan interventions in a general manner, and specifies the types of theories needed to design and implement particular interventions.

Conceptual Frameworks and Nursing Administration

Conceptual frameworks can serve as guides to planning organizational structures in health care agencies. Once a framework has been selected, the nursing administrator can organize nursing services according to the specifications of the framework. As in education, the framework provides the structure for the objectives and goals of the organization as well as the levels of nursing practice in that agency. The conceptual framework can also identify areas of nursing specialization (Rogers, 1973).

ANALYSIS AND EVALUATION OF A CONCEPTUAL FRAMEWORK

Clearly, the distinctions between conceptual frameworks and theories are sufficiently great to warrant different levels of analysis and evaluation. The nursing literature contains such excellent presentations of criteria for theories that further effort in the direction seems unnecessary (Ellis, 1968; Hardy, 1978; Torres & Yura, 1975). The literature also includes evaluative schemata that reflect the confusion between conceptual frameworks and theories. The one initially proposed by Riehl and Roy (1980) used the Dickoff and James (1968) survey list for situation producing theory, and therefore, from the position taken here, is too concrete for abstract conceptual frameworks. Conversely, two other review systems claimed to be designed for theory evaluation but were applied to conceptual frameworks. Both the Duffey and Muhlenkamp (1974) and the Stevens (1979) plans include some questions appropriate to a framework's level of abstraction but, like the Riehl and Roy schema, offer other items more germane to concrete theories. Two additional schema are appropriate for conceptual framework evaluation but seem too limited for comprehensive reviews. Johnson's (1974) criteria are focused solely on social decisions, while Peterson's (1977) questions lack necessary scope and detail. Taken together, however, these several plans provided some building blocks for the construction of the analysis and evaluation plan to be presented here.

The present plan separates questions dealing with analysis from those more appropriate to evaluation. The former queries permit nonjudgmental, detailed examination of the conceptual framework, including its philosophical base, content, and scope. In contrast, evaluative questions allow one to draw judgmental conclusions by focusing on the internal validity of the framework. Both sets of questions lead to a decision to retain, modify, or discard the framework and provide an answer to the pragmatic question of whether I can use the conceptual framework for my nursing activities.

Questions for Analysis

A conceptual framework is derived from its author's personal philosophy and scientific orientation. This philosophic base and the method of framework development (often inductive but sometimes deductive) are often revealed in the author's earlier writings and in preliminary versions of the framework. The first aspect of analysis, then, asks the following questions:

What is the historical evolution of the conceptual framework?
What approach to development of nursing knowledge does the framework exemplify?

It was established earlier that a conceptual framework comprises a set of concepts and linking assumptions, and that the essential concepts of any nursing framework are person, environment, health, and nursing. These components lead to the second aspect of analysis. The questions are:

How are the four essential concepts of nursing explicated in the framework?
—How is person defined and described?
—How is environment defined and described?
—How is health defined? How are wellness and illness differentiated?
—How is nursing defined? What is the goal of nursing? How is the nursing process described?
What statements are made about the relationships among the four concepts?

The final aspect of analysis derives from the fact that any framework must be limited in scope; it cannot deal with all things in the universe. Although most authors begin with the same view of the general purpose of nursing, in their final form nursing frameworks reflect different views of the essential concepts and thus consider different problems in the person-environment interactions related to health. Moreover, the source of these problems may vary. Borrowing from Duffey and Muhlenkamp (1974, p. 571), the questions to be raised are:

—With what problems is the conceptual framework concerned?
—What is the source of these problems?

Questions for Evaluation

The first aspect of evaluation concerns the philosophic underpinnings of the framework. The question is:

—Are the biases and values underlying the conceptual framework explicit?

The next aspect of evaluation deals with the content of the framework and relates back to the answers supplied by the second aspect of analysis. Here the questions to be posed are:

—Does the conceptual framework provide complete descriptions of all four essential concepts of nursing?

—Do the basic assumptions completely link the four concepts?

This second portion of the evaluation must also consider the logic of the framework; its internal structure must be evaluated for congruity. Internal consistency also takes the classification of frameworks into account. Nursing's conceptual frameworks have been categorized according to the discipline of anthropology from which they were derived and are most often labeled developmental, interaction, or systems frameworks. Each of these world views has distinct characteristics that shape the organization of knowledge and methodologies for application. Internal consistency is especially important if the framework incorporates more than one view of any of the essential concepts, since each has different criteria for determining the truth of statements. A synthesis that mixes perspectives also mixes truth criteria. However, it is possible to translate viewpoints by redefining concepts in a consistent manner. Translation represents the construction of a brand-new unmixed logical framework (Reese & Overton, 1970). The questions to be raised, then, are:

—Is the internal structure of the conceptual framework logically consistent?
—Does the conceptual framework reflect the characteristics of its category type?
—Do the components of the conceptual framework reflect logical translation of diverse perspectives?

Johnson's (1974, p. 376) evaluation criteria represent another aspect for consideration. She maintained that conceptual frameworks are validated by social decisions. The first is social congruence, and the question is:

—Does the conceptual framework lead to nursing activities that meet social expectations or do the expectations created by the framework require societal changes?

The second decision is social significance, and here the question is:

—Does the conceptual framework lead to nursing actions that make important differences in the client's health status?

The third decision is social utility, and the question to be raised is:

—Is the conceptual framework comprehensive enough to provide general guides for practice, research, education, and administration?

The third part of evaluation reflects the relation between conceptual frameworks and theories. As noted earlier, theories are derived from frameworks; thus, the theory generating contributions of the conceptual framework should be judged. The result of any known empirical tests of the derived theories also is to be evaluated. The questions to be posed are:

—Does the conceptual framework generate empirically testable theories?
—Do tests of derived theories yield evidence in support of the framework?

The final aspect of evaluation is as general as the frameworks themselves. This question judges the contribution of the framework to nursing knowledge, asking:

—What is the overall contribution of this conceptual framework to the body of nursing knowledge?

This plan for analysis and evaluation of conceptual frameworks of nursing assists nurses to compare various models prior to choosing one as the guideline for their endeavors. It is imperative, however, that the reader understand on what level conceptual frameworks may be compared. The analysis and evaluation of conceptual frameworks allows one to draw conclusions about the internal validity of each, but not to make external comparisons among different frameworks. This important distinction implies "that any conceptual model is valid insofar as it is reasonably sound with regard to the particular anthropology employed (that is, man as developing, adapting, interacting)" (Zbilut, 1978, p. 128). Since models explicate the phenomena of distinct disciplines or schools of thought, direct comparisons cannot be made. Reese and Overton (1970) cautioned that "because of basic lack of communication, the partial overlap in subject matter, and the difference in truth criteria, [each framework] must be evaluated separately, and in obedience to its own ground rules" (p. 122). Thus, judgments are limited to the adequacy and internal validity of each conceptual framework as it stands alone. External comparisons are therefore limited to such issues as the completeness or social consequences of one framework versus another.

An analysis of the conceptual framework of nursing constructed by the University of Connecticut School of Nursing faculty will be presented in Chapter 3 and an evaluation of that framework will be discussed in Chapter 12.

3

The Crisis Theory Conceptual Framework

Eileen Murphy
Jacqueline Fawcett

This chapter describes the development of the crisis theory conceptual framework for the curriculum of the University of Connecticut School of Nursing and is organized according to the criteria for analysis of conceptual frameworks of nursing presented in Chapter 2. These criteria are stated in the following questions.

1. What is the historical evolution of the conceptual framework? What approach to development of nursing knowledge does the framework exemplify?
2. How are the four essential concepts of nursing explicated in the framework?
   How is person defined and described?
   How is environment defined and described?
   How is health defined? How are wellness and illness differentiated?
   How is nursing defined? What is the goal of nursing? How is the nursing process described?
3. With what problems is the conceptual framework concerned? What is the source of these problems?

As noted in Chapter 2, a conceptual framework that is to be used for a curriculum must include ideas about the discipline of nursing; about person, environment, health, and nursing; about education; and about the teaching-learning process. This chapter focuses on the development of content related to the discipline and to the four essential concepts of nursing. Later chapters will describe organization

of courses and course content, teaching strategies, and class and
clinical laboratory settings.

DEVELOPMENT OF THE
CONCEPTUAL FRAMEWORK

When the faculty of the University of the Connecticut School of Nursing
began planning a new curriculum, very little was to be found in the
nursing literature relating to the construction and use of conceptual
frameworks. The faculty had some rather vague and abstract ideas
about the need for a conceptual framework to unify and organize
course offerings, but most faculty members were unaware of the specific and concrete functions provided by a framework. Furthermore,
the faculty was relatively uninformed about the components of a
framework for a curriculum and about how such a framework could
be constructed. Consequently, mistakes were made and frustrations
and disappointments experienced. Finally, however, all the excitement and satisfactions of creating something new, different, and useful were felt.

Initial Assumptions

The faculty's early efforts toward preparing for change have been
described by White and Coburn (1977). This work led to formulation
of assumptions about the nature of a new curriculum. The faculty
agreed that the curriculum would feature an integrated approach to
the organization of nursing content; that the nursing major would be
concentrated in the upper division, or the last two years of the four-
year baccalaureate program; that a team-teaching approach would be
used in nursing courses; that School of Nursing faculty would teach
nursing content while prerequisite and supporting content would be
taught by other members of the university community in non-nursing
courses; that the nursing process would be used to organize certain
aspects of nursing content; and that a theoretical formulation would
be used to describe and organize all aspects of nursing content.

Development of the Philosophy of Nursing
and Nursing Education

Early work on the new curriculum included development of a statement of philosophy that described the faculty's beliefs, attitudes, and

values related to nursing and nursing education—a relatively innocuous document that represents the commonly held ideas of most nurse educators. However, the development of this statement stimulated much controversy and many heated, lengthy debates among faculty members. Since the philosophy symbolized the first irrevocable step in the process of change, these reactions were both inevitable and essential (Bennis, Benne, & Chin, 1976). Many anxieties, hostilities, and personality conflicts arose in the faculty, often masked as concerns about the philosophy. The time devoted to these controversies and concerns proved to be extremely helpful in facilitating the change process by providing an early opportunity for faculty members to advance their viewpoints, to determine how much attention would be given to each individual's ideas and concerns, and to generally assess which way the winds of change were blowing. Faculty members were thus given a chance to see what the future might hold and to decide whether or not to become part of that change.

The philosophy encompassed beliefs and values that exercised considerable influence over the way the new curriculum was to be constructed. First, the curriculum would include a strong emphasis on nursing in wellness situations as well as in those comprising illness experiences. Second, the curriculum would emphasize a client-centered approach to nursing as opposed to a problem-centered approach. Third, while the curriculum would prepare the student to function independently in a variety of settings, emphasis would also be placed upon the collaborative activities of the nurse as a member of the health team. The beliefs about the process and goals of baccalaureate education in nursing expressed within the philosophy also helped to determine the nature of the evolving curriculum.

Development of Objectives

The next task for the faculty was to operationalize the philosophy through the derivation of program objectives. Since the conceptual framework had not yet been developed, the objectives that resulted from this effort were, as might be expected, global in scope and vague in character (Chater, 1975). Small groups of faculty members were then formed to develop the objectives further. Each group was assigned two program objectives and was charged with the responsibility of formulating as many operational level subobjectives as necessary to ensure that the more global objectives could be measured. Each group then presented its work to the total faculty for discussion, revision, and approval. When all objectives were accepted, they were categorized into levels that described behaviors for each of the years of the nursing major.

The program objectives and subobjectives were written at various levels of abstraction, some in behavioral terms, some not, reflecting differing levels of faculty expertise operating at the time. It was important to learn at that stage that while the end product was neither smooth nor perfect it was serviceable, that further polishing would have been counterproductive at that time. It was understood that more specific and detailed objectives for courses, units, and classes would be derived from the subobjectives, after the conceptual framework had been developed. This was the first task that led to a sense of accomplishment among the faculty and, for some, a beginning sense of excitement about the possibilities suggested by the specific objectives.

Formulation of the Conceptual Framework

As the philosophy and objectives were being developed, faculty members proposed many different theoretical formulations to serve as the basis for the conceptual framework. These were argued at length without consensus. Finally, two faculty members who considered crisis theory to be the best choice of the formulations thus far advanced spent a great deal of time and effort promoting its acceptance Their efforts included distribution of article reprints and excerpts from books, development of position papers explaining crisis theory and its uses in nursing (Koehne & Fawcett, 1971 and 1972), and presentation of a workshop to discuss crisis theory and its merits as an appropriate formulation for the new curriculum. These people were able to sell crisis theory to the faculty because of their own enthusiasm, their knowledge of the formulation, and their ability to suggest concrete ways in which it could be used.

In retrospect it seems clear that much non-productive and time-consuming discussion could have been avoided if small groups had assumed the task of doing for other formulations what these two faculty members had done for crisis theory. Faculty could then have debated the relative merits of each on the basis of increased knowledge and might perhaps have arrived at a decision much sooner.

Even after selecting crisis theory as the theoretical formulation on which to base the conceptual framework, some faculty members had difficulty with the term "crisis" which they equated with ideas of catastrophe or disaster. Because of this negative connotation, many people thought this formulation was too limiting and feared that it would result in a curriculum that was illness-oriented, clearly not in keeping with the faculty's beliefs about wellness as expressed in the philosophy.

The definition finally agreed upon was derived from the work of Caplan and his colleagues (1965) and reflects the connotation of crisis as a turning point, a response to a decisive event signifying danger or opportunity. Crisis is viewed as the impact of any event that challenges the assumed state and forces the individual to change his view of, or readapt to, the world, himself, or both. "Specifically, a crisis is a state of disequilibrium overpowering the individual's homeostatic mechanisms" (Parad & Caplan, 1965, p. 56).

A glossary of terms was developed by the faculty to avoid further misunderstandings about the various concepts of the conceptual framework. This glossary was helpful in the faculty's discussions as the development of the framework continued, and is now used for orientation of new faculty members and students to the school's conceptual framework.

As development of the conceptual framework progressed, the faculty recognized the need to develop comprehensive descriptions of each component of a framework that is to be used for a curriculum. Small groups of faculty members were therefore assigned to develop descriptions of the discipline of nursing, man, education, the teaching-learning process, and the educational setting that would be useful in decision making about curricular components. For example, a comprehensive description of the educational setting identified the institutional factors within the University of Connecticut and the constraints found within the broader community that would have direct influence on the various tasks associated with development and implementation of the curriculum (Heineman, 1973).

Once the faculty had accepted the crisis theory formulation as a basis for the conceptual framework, a small group of faculty members was assigned the task of exploring how crisis theory could be used for curriculum development in general and for development of specific courses as well. A flow chart (adapted from Aguilera and Messick, 1970) of the major ideas contained in the crisis theory formulation was developed (Figure 3-1) to provide a concrete basis for discussion and a common understanding of the events surrounding development and resolution of a crisis. The capitalized terms in Figure 3-1 represent those major ideas. The remainder of this chapter analyzes the conceptual framework according to the criteria for

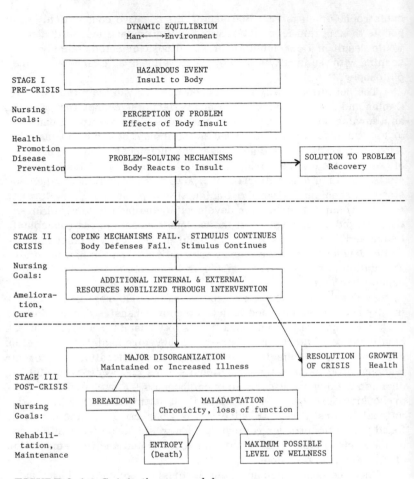

FIGURE 3-1. Crisis theory model.

analysis presented in Chapter 2 and describes the adaptation and expansion of the crisis theory formulation for the conceptual framework of the University of Connecticut School of Nursing.

ANALYSIS OF THE CONCEPTUAL FRAMEWORK

Historical Evolution of the Conceptual Framework

An examination of the historical evolution of a conceptual formulation offers important insights into the philosophical beliefs and pragmatic concerns that influenced its development. Such insights help to clarify questions of meaning and intent not always made clear in the formulation itself.

Although Gerald Caplan's name is most commonly associated with crisis theory, it was Erich Lindemann, another psychiatrist, who developed the rudiments of crisis theory in what he termed "a conceptual frame of reference" for investigating emotional crises. Lindemann (1956) explained that, during the 1940s, he and a number of other psychiatrists were dissatisfied with the prevailing treatment modalities for mental disorders because they emphasized therapy only after illness had developed and often resulted in institutionalization. In seeking an alternative to this medical model, they turned to social scientists and public health workers. The result of this interdisciplinary collaboration was a commitment to develop therapeutic modalities focusing on the maintenance of mental health and the prevention of mental illness. Thus, it is clear that even before the earliest formulations of crisis theory were explicated, the maintenance of mental health and the prevention of mental illness were viewed as legitimate goals for mental health workers.

Lindemann's classic description of bereavement responses of survivors and families of victims of the Coconut Grove nightclub fire in Boston (Lindemann, 1944) is generally accepted as the beginning of crisis theory (Darbonne, 1968). Lindemann made two observations which became the foundation for his subsequent development of preventive mental health programs. The first of these was that psychopathological sequelae to bereavement were less likely to develop when the individual completed an identifiable course of grief resolution. The second was that professional and community caretakers could intervene to help sufferers to mourn adequately (Lindemann, 1944). He hypothesized that these findings could be generalized beyond the bereavement experience to other hazards to psychological well-being. These ideas were translated into clinical practice by Lindemann and his colleagues at the Wellesley Human Relations Service, a community-based mental health program established in 1948 and designed to focus on prevention of mental illness (Caplan, 1964).

In 1956 Lindemann described what he termed a "conceptual framework" for preventive mental health that he had developed from his clinical experiences. This paper contains many of the basic ideas of crisis theory as we know it today. Based upon his observations, Lindemann noted that the occurrence of hazardous events in the lives of individuals has the potential for causing impairment if

not adequately mastered and that these events become crises for
people whose emotional resources are taxed beyond their usual adaptive limits. He noted also that, at times of crisis, individuals are
particularly receptive to helpful advice from mental health workers
(Lindemann, 1956).

In the 1950s Lindemann was joined in his work both at the
Wellesley Human Relations Service and in the Community Mental
Health Program at the Harvard School of Public Health by Gerald
Caplan, another psychiatrist convinced of the efficacy of a public
health approach for the prevention of illness and for the optimum utilization of psychotherapeutic workers. Caplan was struck also by the
role that could be played by other community members in such programs (Caplan, 1951). These concerns are evident in Caplan's
writings, which have expanded the original crisis theory formulation
developed by Lindemann by investigating situations that are potentially crisis-producing, for example, the diagnosis of tuberculosis in
a family member (Parad & Caplan, 1965) and the reactions of parents
to the birth of a premature infant (Caplan, et al., 1965). Associates
of Lindemann and Caplan used the crisis theory framework to investigate possible interventions during potentially crisis producing situations (Parad, 1965). Caplan also used commonalities he found
among his own work, that of his Harvard colleagues, and that of other
investigators of crisis behavior, the crisis process, and precipitating
factors (Caplan, 1965) to formulate the empirical generalizations of
crisis theory.

Meanwhile, American consumers and providers alike were finding traditional mental health services for families, groups, and communities to be time-consuming, expensive, and frequently ineffective
In 1963, at the urging of the Kennedy administration, Congress passed
the Community Mental Health Centers Act, which provided for the
development of comprehensive community mental health programs
that would emphasize prevention as well as treatment (Darbonne,
1968). However, guidance and direction were needed for such community-based preventive efforts.

Caplan's 1964 book, Principles of Preventive Psychiatry, presented a set of suggested guidelines for the development of these new
community-based programs. In presenting his proposal for primary
prevention, Caplan explicated his version of crisis theory. Like
Lindemann's original work, this version noted the crisis-producing
potential inherent in certain events faced by individuals during the
course of their lives. Unlike the earlier work, however, Caplan
emphasized that appropriate interventions could not only prevent

illness but could promote mental health. In fact, Caplan asserted that the intervention received was a more important determinant of the outcome of a crisis than were the antecedent conditions or the personal characteristics of the individual experiencing the crisis (Caplan, 1964). Caplan's approach included two other important points. First, crisis was viewed as a time-limited phenomenon, usually resolved for better or worse in a relatively short period of time. Second, during the disequilibrium of crisis, the individual was seen as more susceptible to the influence of others than during periods of stability (Caplan, 1964). Thus, Caplan expanded Lindemann's ideas to include a more detailed description of the crisis process and to emphasize the characteristics and effects of intervention.

Caplan's influence on the development of mental health programs can be inferred from the multitude of crisis intervention programs that are offered in almost every community. The crisis theory framework has been used by a variety of disciplines to identify many experiences for which intensive, short-term interventions are expected to be effective in preventing mental illness.

Although most health professionals have some knowledge of crisis theory, a review of pertinent literature reveals many misconceptions and misunderstandings about the substance and intent of the original formulation. Therefore, a summary of crisis theory as it was developed by its originators (Lindemann, 1944, 1956; Caplan, 1951, 1961, 1964) is presented here.

Summary of the Crisis Theory Formulation

During his life span, the individual encounters many situations that have the potential for upsetting his steady state. These situations are termed hazardous events and are divided into two categories. The first category, termed developmental or normative, encompasses all maturational stages and the developmental tasks required for each. Examples of developmental hazardous events might be birth, weaning, school entry, marriage. The second classification, termed situational hazardous events, includes only accidental occurrences within the life of the individual. Examples of situational hazardous events might be the loss or change of jobs, relocation, addition of family member, loss of a significant other. These deviations in the steady state are thought to arise from within the individual, from the environment, or from both.

Stage I. For an event to have potential for crisis, the individual must perceive the alteration in his steady state to be a problem, which then results in his experiencing heightened tension and evokes known problem-solving behaviors. If the problem-solving behaviors are adequate to deal with the event, solution of the problem occurs and no crisis develops. The individual returns to a state of equilibrium.

Stage II. If, however, the individual's usual problem-solving mechanisms are inadequate to solve the problem in an expected period of time, he moves into a state of crisis. The individual must see the situation as constituting an important problem for him that he cannot escape or solve with his habitual problem-solving resources. It must be emphasized here that the original formulations are very clear that the development of a crisis is dependent upon the unique reaction of the individual to the event and is not inherent in the event itself. Nor is it determined by the amount of hazard perceived in the event by another observer.

Four phases have been identified as the components of the crisis experience. The first has already been described as the problem-solving effort. The second stage occurs when problem-solving attempts are unsuccessful. This results in a further rise in tension and feelings of helplessness, ineffectuality, anxiety, fear, guilt, shame. If the stimulus continues, the third stage follows, characterized by a further increase in tension which serves to stimulate the mobilization of additional internal and external resources. During this stage the individual may engage in trial and error attempts to solve the problem; he may call upon emergency problem-solving techniques; he may redefine the problem in some way amenable to solution; he may resign himself to the loss of certain goals; he may use perceptual distortion; he may actively give up. The present crisis may also evoke memories of old problems whose unsatisfactory resolution may add to the present burden.

Because of the disorganization and the resulting loss of defense mechanisms, it is at this stage that the individual in crisis is said to be most open to outside intervention. In fact, he often solicits help from others during this phase. The expanded version of crisis theory (Caplan, 1964) places much emphasis on the importance of the help offered by a significant other at this point. It is stated that the quality of the intervention can easily tip the balance toward health or illness, and is probably a more powerful determinant of the outcome of the crisis than are such antecedent factors as the nature of the hazard or the past experiences of the individual.

Stage III. If crisis resolution is successful, the individual learns new problem-solving behaviors and therefore returns to a steady state that is at a higher level of functioning than that which he experienced before the crisis occurred. The crisis theorists have asserted that it is possible to increase an individual's resistance to mental disorders by helping him to extend his repertoire of effective problem-solving skills. It is this potential for growth that crisis theorists claim is one of the major factors that serve to distinguish crisis from stress which is said to have only psychopathological potential.

A second factor that distinguishes crisis from stress is that the former is time-limited. Although the exact time frame for a crisis is not known, there is general agreement that a state of crisis will most likely be resolved in one way or another within six weeks of its onset.

Even in cases where the crisis has not been resolved in a growth-producing manner, some kind of resolution must take place. This may be an unhealthy adjustment, lowering the level of functioning and increasing one's vulnerability to mental disorders. The fourth phase of the crisis experience is reached when no resolution can occur, tension mounts to the breaking point, and major disorganization of the individual results.

The Crisis Theory Model

This summary of crisis theory demonstrates its usefulness for prevention of mental illness and promotion of mental health. It is clear, however, that physical-physiological responses to hazardous events are not accounted for. Therefore, given nursing's interest in the total person (Donaldson & Crowley, 1978), and the faculty's explicitly stated belief in the person as a biological, psychological, social, and cultural being (Kennedy & Collins, 1974), the crisis theory formulation had to be extended to the biophysical realm in order to be useful for the curriculum.

The faculty reasoned that a biophysical stimulus, or hazardous event, could provoke the psychosocial responses described above. They further reasoned that a similar process involving analogous phases could be described for biophysical responses to hazardous events. Thus, it became possible to talk of physiological as well as psychological disequilibrium and resolution of upsets in the steady state. The biophysical responses to hazardous events were added to the original flow chart (lower case captions under the capitalized headings in Figure 3-1).

One area of concern with this postulated extension of crisis theory to the biophysical realm is the growth factor. In some biophysical problems growth may be seen in the development of compensatory processes as the body's response to crisis. These responses are not found in all situations however. In fact, sometimes the body must function at a lower level of wellness than it did before crisis, even when intervention is judged successful. Using a holistic approach, it may be possible to show growth in some aspect of the individual's functioning, even in the face of reduced biophysical health, but that does not address the particular concern in question. Therefore, the application of this formulation to biophysical problems does not constitute a perfect fit. However, it remains a useful way of identifying and organizing relevant phenomena in such situations.

Approach to Framework Development
Exemplified by the Model

The original crisis theory formulation was based on inductive modes of thought and focused primarily on identification of components of the crisis experience, while the later version included attention to promoting mental health and added emphasis on various aspects of crisis intervention.

The formulations of crisis theory were used to develop the conceptual framework for the University of Connecticut School of Nursing curriculum. As noted above, the ideas of crisis theory were expanded to include the individual's physiological responses to hazardous events. The conceptual framework thus considers the person in a comprehensive manner. Moreover, as will be explained later in this chapter, the conceptual framework added more extensive ideas about health to the crisis theory formulation and crisis intervention strategies were incorporated into a problem-solving approach to the nursing process. This expansion of the original crisis theory formulation advanced by Lindemann, Caplan, and their colleagues represents a deductive approach to conceptual framework development.

The next section of the chapter presents an overview of the University of Connecticut School of Nursing faculty's translation and incorporation of crisis theory into their ideas about the discipline of nursing and about man. These ideas will be analyzed in relation to nursing's four essential concepts.

Essential Concepts of Nursing

Person. The crisis theory conceptual framework that faculty formulated identifies the person as an integrated biological, psychological, social, and cultural being whose growth and development along a continuum from birth to death reflects order, consistency, and continuity in a normative sense, and whose behavior, therefore, has a certain degree of predictability. The person is viewed as an open system that can live in a state of dynamic equilibrium through constant adaptation to the environment. Each person is thought to have a specific set of needs that motivate the behavior required to maintain equilibrium, and each person has a responsibility for and the freedom to achieve equilibrium through dependent and interdependent interactions with the environment (Kennedy & Collins, 1974).

Throughout life, it is thought that people encounter psychosocial and biophysical hazardous events that have the potential to interfere with their usual ways of dealing with themselves and with the world. As noted earlier, hazardous events are thought to include all maturational events and the sudden, unexpected situations occurring throughout the person's life that represent real, threatened, or imagined loss of dynamic equilibrium (Rapaport, 1965). Thus, hazardous events are classified as developmental or situational, and, when overlapping, as combined developmental-situational hazardous events. The incorporation of these various types of hazardous events into curriculum course content will be discussed in Chapter 4.

Since hazardous events represent real, threatened, or imagined loss to the person, they have been further classified into the following seven major loss categories: loss of relationships; loss of mobility; loss of regulation; loss of patency; loss of protective mechanisms; loss of sensory-motor exchange; and loss of reproductive adequacy. The organization of curriculum content into these loss categories is presented in Chapters 4 and 6. Each person is thought to have an evolving repertoire of coping mechanisms, or problem-solving skills, that facilitates the ability to deal with hazardous events. Moreover, each person has certain internal and external resources actually or potentially available that can be used to augment these coping mechanisms.

These ideas and descriptions of the person can be extended to the family and the community when these are the focal points of nursing care. Moreover, these descriptions of the person apply not only to the consumer of health care but to the learner and the educator as well (Kennedy & Collins, 1974).

Environment. The crisis theory conceptual framework identifies the environment as everything outside the person. This includes family members, friends, coworkers, health care personnel, and other people, as well as organizations and physical objects. As noted above, the environment contains the resources that may be needed to augment the person's innate coping mechanisms. The environment also contains hazardous events that pose threats to the person's dynamic equilibrium, as well as those factors that put certain individuals at risk for development of crises.

Health. Health is viewed as a continuum from high-level wellness to illness. Halbert Dunn's (1959) idea of health as a function of the relationship between the person and the environment has been incorporated into the crisis theory conceptual framework. According to Dunn,

> high-level wellness for the individual is defined as an integrated method of functioning which is oriented toward maximizing the potential of which the individual is capable. It requires that the individual maintain a continuum of balance and purposeful direction within the environment where he is functioning (p. 4).

According to the crisis theory conceptual framework, people are also assessed when they are in a state of dynamic equilibrium with their environments. This means that their coping mechanisms are completely adequate to meet and master the challenges posed by hazardous events.

People move away from high-level wellness and toward the illness end of the continuum when their usual coping mechanisms are not completely sufficient to overcome the threats posed by the hazardous events. Exact placement on the continuum is based on the person's perception of the severity of the hazardous event, adequacy of the person's coping mechanisms, available resources, and ability to use resources. Being in a state of disequilibrium, or crisis, does not automatically lead to an assessment of illness. In fact, people are considered to be most seriously ill when they have experienced an unsuccessful resolution of the crisis, that is, are maladapting.

A special feature of the crisis theory conceptual framework is the explication of events following the occurrence of crisis. As noted earlier, people are more open to intervention and more susceptible to intervention efforts during the crisis period. If intervention is effective, the crisis is resolved and high-level wellness is regained. It is thought that successful resolution of a crisis, which is postulated to occur within six weeks, results in growth of the person. This is usually manifested by increased coping mechanisms, that is, increased ability to solve problems or overcome hazardous events before they are perceived as crises.

If intervention is not effective, or if it is not sought during the crisis period, major disorganization or illness is thought to follow. This can be manifested by such psychosocial and/or biophysical maladaptation as chronic illness and can be resolved as maintenance of the maximum possible level of wellness, as continued maladaptation, or as death.

Nursing. The primary goal of nursing in the crisis theory conceptual framework is to foster high-level wellness. Secondary goals have been developed by the faculty and related to a conceptualization of crisis as a series of three stages (see figure 3-1).

In Stage I, Pre-Crisis, the goals are health promotion and disease prevention. These goals are appropriate when the person has adequate coping mechanisms to overcome the threats posed by hazardous events. Health promotion is accomplished by enhancing the dynamic equilibrium between the person and environment through such intervention strategies as anticipatory guidance and ego strengthening or general support (Caplan, 1964). When disease prevention is the goal, interventions emphasize augmentation of the person's repertoire of coping mechanisms and/or reduction of the hazardous potential of specific events.

In Stage II, Crisis, the nursing goal is amelioration or cure. Here reduction of the impact of the hazardous event is facilitated by interventions that focus on mobilizing internal and external resources.

In Stage III, Post-Crisis, goals include rehabilitation, maintenance of an optimal level of health, and support through the process of dying. Rehabilitation focuses on support of the person through the final stages of convalescence to healthy resolution of the crisis, with emphasis on enhancing growth. Interventions include measures that reverse or lessen effects of breakdown, maladaptation, and chronicity. Maintenance of an optimal level of health is appropriate when chronic illness cannot be avoided. Here, interventions may take the form of anticipatory guidance, general support, and mobilization of available internal and external resources. Finally, if death is inevitable, the goal of support through the dying process is appropriate.

The crisis theory conceptual framework identifies the nursing process as a four step problem-solving activity encompassing assessment, planning, intervention, and evaluation. Since the framework emphasizes the importance of the person's coping mechanisms, existing resources, and perceptions of events, assessment focuses on identification of these factors in both psychosocial and biophysical realms. Planning emphasizes priority setting and identification of appropriate nursing goals in collaboration with clients and in keeping with their perceptions of events. Interventions are based upon the four main categories outlined by Caplan (1964): ego strengthening or general support; mobilizing environmental sources of support; anticipatory guidance; and help in specific crises. Evaluation considers the state of the dynamic equilibrium between the person and the environment following intervention. Here, the current coping mechanisms and resources are assessed, as in person's perception of ability to deal with future hazardous events.

Relationships Among Essential Concepts

The following statements link the concepts of person, environment, health, and nursing.

1. Dynamic equilibrium describes the open system in which the person interacts with the environment during periods of high-level wellness. The goal of nursing is to promote and maintain this dynamic equilibrium.

2. Hazardous events have the potential for disruption of the dynamic equilibrium between person and environment, and thus, disruption of the state of high-level wellness. Personal and environmental factors affect the person's perception of the impact of hazardous events. Coping mechanisms are used by the person to prevent or deal with a crisis. These problem-solving methods facilitate the person's adaptation to environmental changes which affect health. The goal of nursing is to promote accurate perception of events in order to maintain the highest level of wellness possible.

Nurses assess the effectiveness of current coping mechanisms and the resources available to augment these coping mechanisms.

3. A crisis occurs when the person's coping mechanisms are inadequate in maintaining a dynamic person-environment equilibrium. The goal of nursing is to ameliorate or cure the effects of disruption in the steady state.

4. Resolution of a crisis requires additional resources to assist the person regain a dynamic equilibrium with the environment. Nurses help the person to identify and use these resources. Successful resolution results in the return of the person to a state of wellness. Unsuccessful resolution results in continued illness or death. The goal of nursing is to promote the maximum possible level of wellness regardless of the type of crisis resolution.

Problems Considered by the Conceptual Framework

It should be obvious by now that the crisis theory conceptual framework is concerned with people's perceptions of and responses to disruptions in the dynamic equilibrium with their environments. The sources of these disruptions are developmental, situational, or combined developmental-situational hazardous events.

CONCLUSION

The crisis theory conceptual framework is congruent with the values and beliefs expressed in the school's statement of philosophy. Since emphasis is placed upon the individual's previously learned coping behaviors, upon his existing or available strengths and resources, and upon his unique perceptions and reactions, it emphasizes the client-centered, individualized approach to nursing practice. Since the focus of crisis theory is upon the strengths and resources that the individual has, those that he needs, and those that he gains through successful resolution of crisis, the major emphasis of the formulation is wellness oriented. Because the formulation addresses those events, normative or accidental, that make up life, it deals with the total life process rather than just periods of stress or illness. Because growth following successful resolution of the crisis is a salient feature of the formulation, it supports a wellness-illness-wellness viewpoint. Finally, the mobilization of resources in all stages often demands the participation of many kinds and levels of health workers, thus providing opportunities for the nurse to function interdependently as a health team member.

4

Organization
of the Nursing Major

Dorothy Coburn

Utilization of the conceptual framework was not easy. For one reason, very few faculty had as clear an understanding of the concepts and their relationships as the descriptions presented in Chapter 3. These understandings were gradually developed and clarified as the framework was operationalized. Moreover, faculty were accustomed to teaching without a conceptual framework or with individual, poorly-defined frameworks; now they had to adapt to a specified framework with which to design an integrated nursing curriculum. The conceptual framework stood the test and assisted faculty to make rational decisions about general and specific aspects of the nursing major.

DESIGN OF THE NURSING MAJOR

An upper division major involves a four semester plan. Within this plan, consideration had to be given to theory courses, process courses, and supportive courses. Components of the conceptual framework (that is, theories of education, man, crisis, and nursing process) readily prescribed the sequence of these courses. Guidance was also provided by the philosophy which states, "Learning activities proceed from the simple to the complex and from singular tasks to integrative activities." (University of Connecticut School of Nursing, 1977, p. 40).

Hazardous events (a major concept of the crisis model) lend themselves to a simple to complex learning sequence. Developmental hazardous events are predictable and have been validated in the literature—they are viewed as a normal and healthy process in the growth of human beings. Situational hazardous events are not predictable and vary extensively in terms of the degree of threat to or risk for the client. When a situational hazardous event occurs in combination with a developmental hazardous event, the impact on the client is greater and produces more disorganization of the client, demanding more sophisticated and integrative knowledge and skills from the nurse. Thus, hazardous events prescribe the progression from simple to complex.

The nursing process is another component of the conceptual framework that had a major influence on sequence, specifically in the development of the process courses. The theory of man, a holistic view, blended well with crisis theory and the nursing process. A detailed description of theory and process courses will be presented later in this chapter and the relationship of concepts should become clearer to the reader at that time.

Changing from a semi-traditional nursing curriculum to an integrated curriculum presented many problems. Early in this process of change, a content development group was organized. All clinical specialty areas were represented in this group, and one of its initial tasks was to develop and organize a list of concepts essential to the nursing curriculum. The process of this activity was more important than the product as it assisted faculty to begin to look at the integrative aspects of the curriculum, and it generated dialogue beyond one's small teaching group.

From the content development group, initial plans for the nursing major began to evolve. Two sub-groups each set forth a proposal for the organization of the junior and senior years, one with a wellness-illness focus, the other with an illness-wellness focus. Both groups included rationale, underlying basic assumptions, and a general view of each semester as prescribed by these assumptions and related concepts. The proposals were submitted to the faculty for suggestions, and a faculty meeting day was set aside for presentation and discussion During a summer workshop, the proposed plans were scrutinized in depth, and an independent group presented yet another plan. Issues and rationales were challenged, debated, and defended. The final plan, a wellness-illness-wellness model, emerged from the total faculty group and, although it involved some compromises, the major premises of all were included. This wellness-illness-wellness approach was clearly supported by the conceptual framework. The stages of crisis (pre-crisis, crisis, and post-crisis) are particularly supportive of this sequence.

IDENTIFICATION OF CONTENT

The group process described here—input from faculty to small groups then back to faculty—has been an effective one. The total faculty must be involved in the initial planning phase and in the final decision-making phase; small groups are the most efficient way to accomplish specific tasks.

An early approach to course development that involved several small groups simultaneously attempting to develop a specific course proved to be quite non-productive. Each group had course descriptions and a theoretical framework from which to proceed; only one group, however, was able to accomplish the task. The success of this group can perhaps be attributed to the fact that it was designing the first course in the upper division and that it was dealing with content new to the nursing major. Other groups appeared bogged down by the fact that no faculty decisions had been made about specific content or the progression of content. In this instance, division into small groups took place too soon.

Another issue may have interfered with task accomplishment—faculty did not know how or by what criteria teaching assignments would be made. As a consequence, some faculty felt reluctant to make specific decisions for courses with which they might not be directly involved. The dynamics of this behavior can be related to such other issues as delaying tactics, degree of commitment, decision-making without authority, and academic freedom. Although the teaching assignment issue was not then and is not now considered a major stumbling block, it may be a covert issue that needs to be addressed during a major curriculum revision. A group that creates a course may become possessive of that course, of its content or of teaching responsibilities for it.

Use of Consultants

At various stages of change, external assistance in the form of consultants can be very helpful and is often essential. The use of consultants is an interesting phenomenon in our world today, particularly in academia. When funding is available, one frequently sees a parade of consultants whose areas of expertise may or may not be suitable to the project at hand. Like enjoying a smorgasbord, we try a little of this, a little of that, whether or not we need it. Frequently, we are not selective but try to sample as much as our plates—our minds—can hold. With consultants, as with the smorgasbord, if we go back for seconds, it is for that which was most interesting, most satisfying.

When seeking a consultant or considering honoring a request to consult, it is wise to ask what specific needs the group has and who is the most appropriate person to meet those needs. It may be that these questions cannot be answered. Perhaps the project goal is clear but the means of reaching that goal are not. In such instances, a smorgasbord may be necessary. Whether the consultant is there for an hour or a week, it is extremely important that the participants formally evaluate the experience because this evaluative data can assist future consultants to meet the needs of the group.

One consultant became particularly useful to the University of Connecticut faculty. She was consistently able to excite and challenge. Her own enthusiasm and confidence generated enthusiasm and confidence in others so that even skeptics began moving toward the identified goal. At a time when the faculty was experiencing frustration and lack of accomplishment, her suggestion that a grid be developed provided a great forward thrust.

Developing the Grid

A grid is a blueprint that depicts the content of all associated courses, in this instance, the courses in the nursing major. The final product lists on one sheet of columned paper the theory and process content of the nine nursing courses, and, on another paper, the strands content related to all nursing courses. Vertical columns present the major concepts for individual courses. Reading horizontally, each concept can be traced through a four or five semester sequence (see figure 4-1).

The development of the grid was a remarkable piece of group work. Picture, if you will, twenty-five faculty members, representing a variety of educational and clinical backgrounds and harboring individual and collective vested interests. They are seated in a classroom with stationary and portable blackboards. Their task is to identify all of the content to be taught in the junior and senior nursing courses. As faculty brainstorm ideas for organizing content, the framework provides the pattern. Since loss is a predominant concept in crisis theory, seven loss categories were identified—loss of patency, relationships, regulation, mobility, protective mechanisms, sensory-motor exchange, and reproductive adequacy. The blackboards fill as faculty members call out their suggestions for specific

		Semester 3 or 4 Theory	Semester 5 Theory	Semester 5 Process	Semester 6 Theory	Semester 6 Process	
T h e o r y / P r o c e s s	C O N T E N T						G R I D Page 1
S T A N D A R D	History						G R I D Page 2
	IPR						
	Health Teaching						
C O N T E N T	Research						G R I D Page 3
	Leadership						

FIGURE 4-1. Miniature facsimile of the format of the grid. (The complete grid continues on through semester eight.)

content to be included in each loss category. At the end of each work session, words are transferred to strips of brown paper. What emerges are long lists that are a mix of concepts and medical problems. Later the grid is edited to be more conceptually oriented.

Early in this process, faculty began to allocate content to the junior or senior level. The criteria for making these decisions rested with the conceptual framework and a simple-to-complex sequence. Faculty considered the potential of a hazardous event to precipitate a crisis, including the relationship of a situational hazardous event to a developmental hazardous event, and the degree of complexity and sophistication of the nursing interventions. There were some content areas that related to all nursing courses—these were identified as strands. Ideas for strands emerged as work on courses began. Volunteer groups of three to four faculty members were formed to work on the conceptual development of the strands and report back to the total group. Utilizing the philosophy and objectives of the program, decisions were made regarding the inclusion or exclusion of content as strands. The selected strands were leadership, research, history, interpersonal relationships, and health teaching.

In some nursing programs, each of these strands might be an individual course. The proposal that health teaching be a separate course was rejected as contrary to the concept of integration. Furthermore, it was found that strands promote levels of learning that can be applied to the learner as well as to content.

Concepts from strands were ranked in simple-to-complex order and incorporated primarily in the process courses. This is a logical placement since most of the strand content relates to theory and skills specifically applied in the clinical laboratory. The exception is the history strand, which has been integrated appropriately into both theory and process courses.

With the allocation of content to levels completed, the loss categories became the units in the theory courses. Specific hazardous events were selected to illustrate the concepts and form the basis of class presentations. Faculty agreed that placement of concepts on the grid would remain constant, but illustrative hazardous events might vary from year to year. Figure 6-3 is a segment of the grid which illustrates the organization of content within a loss category. The nursing process was the organizing framework for the process courses, and on the grid one can trace the intellectual, interpersonal, and psychomotor content relative to each step of the process. The leadership strand can be traced through the five semesters beginning with the sophomore course, as illustrated in figure 4-2.

The philosophy of laboratory should be mentioned here as it influenced placement of laboratory activities and was a frequent source of conflict. The process of the development of this philosophy followed the pattern previously described—initial input of total faculty, then discussion by a small group for further development and refinement, and finally, return of the product to faculty for discussion and decision. Since the acceptance of the first, rather lengthy, edition, the philosophy has had two revisions. The need for revisions became

	Semester 3 or 4 NU 150	Semester 5 Nu 208	Semester 6 Nu 228	Semester 7 Nu 238	Semester 7 ID 200	Semester 8 Nu 275	Semester 8 Nu 285
Leadership Strand	Membership in groups Group process Health team membership/ leadership Collegiality Collaboration Bureaucratic/ professional models	Responsi- bility and accounta- bility for own actions Ethics	Nursing team Member- ship Responsi- bility Accounta- bility	Accountabil- ity Outcomes of client care Collabora- tion Self-evalu- ation Health team Membership Responsi- bility Accounta- bility	Shifting leadership within health team	Leadership role in groups Peer review Self-evalu- ation Membership role in groups Peer review Self-evalu- ation	Leadership for group of clients/peers Management Systems of delivery Professional/ bureaucratic conflict Reality Shock Change Evaluation of effect of professional behavior on client, group, peers Health team leadership responsibil- ity accounta- bility

FIGURE 4-2. Leadership strand content (excerpt from grid).

apparent as faculty struggled to apply the philosophy and operationalize the new behaviors described for faculty, students, and agency
personnel. Changes were essentially to correct a perceived rigidity
of language rather than in philosophical issues, although some issues
were frequently debated. Utilization of the philosophy and the corresponding issues will be discussed in Chapter 7.

DESCRIPTION OF THEORY AND PROCESS COURSES

Decisions were not always made in logical sequence; for example,
requirements imposed by catalogue printing made it necessary to
prepare course descriptions long before content was defined. Since
faculty had agreed to utilize crisis theory and the nursing process
as unifying concepts, it was possible to write general descriptions in
language appropriate to these concepts. Following is a description of
specific courses and the rationale for progression and pairing of
these courses.

Although this curriculum is an upper division major, the first
nursing course appears in the sophomore year. Essentially, it is a
socialization course, designed to explore philosophies and common
perceptions of nursing. Perceptions are validated as students explore the role of the nurse as a member of th health team and the
trends and issues related to the profession. The course also intro-
duces the student to the philosophy and conceptual framework of the
curriculum and includes content in each of the five strands. Placement of this course in the lower division provides the student an
opportunity to reexamine career goals before making a commitment
to the upper division major.

In the first semester of the upper division, the focus is on health.
The theory course, "Man and Health—A Study of Continua," details
those concepts pertaining to health maintenance and promotion; the
process course, "Assessment in Levels of Health," attends to assessment. Essentially, the theory course focuses on the pre-crisis state
from birth to death with an emphasis on developmental hazardous
events and the intrinsic and extrinsic factors which affect man's
potential for health and his life-coping mechanisms. The process
course examines wellness through physical and psychological assessments.

The process course includes a laboratory component. In the
college laboratory, the student acquires the assessment skills to be
utilized in the clinical laboratory. Clinically, the student interacts

with healthy persons in day care centers, senior citizen centers, schools, prenatal clinics, newborn nurseries, and postpartum units. During this semester students follow a pregnant couple through the prenatal, delivery and postpartum experience.

Also in this semester, the family study begins. Some students continue with the family mentioned above, others are assigned families from within the university community and some are obtained from other sources. This relationship with the family continues through the senior year. The student is expected to make monthly visits during the academic year and to engage in activities such as health history, developmental tests, health teaching, and neighborhood assessment. The emphasis is always on health and the promotion of existing strengths and resources. Problems associated with the implementation of the family study were related to logistics, faculty utilization (of the family), and student motivation.

Because in any given year between 200 and 225 healthy families are being followed by students, logistical problems are enormous. The initial recruitment of families was from the university's employee association and the retiree's association. A large percentage of the participating families came from the latter group and, consequently, provided the student with a somewhat restricted view of the life cycle. Students are now responsible for finding their own families—this appears to be a more efficient process of recruitment.

The faculty's utilization of and commitment to the family study was initially highly individualized. Although everyone theoretically endorsed the value of the study, priorities were usually established by pressure factors. Adaptations demanded of faculty in terms of classroom and laboratory teaching took time and energy and, for some, required major adjustments. Faculty expectations and responsibilities toward the family study were poorly defined and so assumed a low priority. Once faculty became more comfortable in other areas, and once a committee composed of faculty representatives from the junior and senior levels was organized to coordinate the logistical and clinical aspects of the family study, the individual faculty member's role became more structured.

Maintaining student motivation has been and continues to be a concern. Once students have completed health assessments, they frequently have difficulty identifying objectives for visits. A majority of undergraduate students find the glamour and challenge to be in illness, not in health. Most students do develop an interest in their families, however, and, with faculty guidance and support, can continue to learn about levels of wellness through the utilization of resources and adaptive coping mechanisms employed by these families.

In the sixth semester the students move into the illness portion of the health continuum. The theory course, "Manifestations of Health Crises," continues a study of crisis theory through an examination of situational hazardous events. The situational events are described in terms of bio-psycho-social concepts as they relate to the major health problems encountered by man. Specific hazardous events are selected as the basis for class presentations.

The process course, "Planning and Intervention in Levels of Health," focuses on these two phases of the nursing process; intellectual skills are addressed in the classroom, psychomotor skills in the college laboratory. In the clinical laboratory, students use their assessment skills to gather data about persons who are encountering situational hazardous events. Planning and intervention follows in selected developmental and situational crises.

Three supportive courses run concurrently with the junior-year nursing courses. In the health-focused semester, students take a nutritional science course and, in the sixth semester, pathobiology. These courses are taught by their respective departments in the university. In addition, a two semester pharmacology course, offered by the school of pharmacy, is required.

In the senior year, the teaching-learning becomes more complex as the student is called upon to integrate previous learning with new knowledge and skills. In the seventh semester theory course, "Crises and their Resolution," emphasis is on life-coping mechanisms associated with a crisis that has both situational and developmental components. In essence, those events selected for study have a strong potential to precipitate a crisis. To complete the crisis cycle, post-crisis resolutions, both adaptive and maladaptive, are considered.

In the process course, "Intervention and Evaluation in Levels of Health," the cycle of the nursing process is completed with emphasis on evaluation and new learning related to intervention. In the clinical laboratory the total nursing process is applied to crisis situations and their aftermaths.

The non-nursing course required this semester is an interdepartmental course which provides an interdisciplinary approach to health care and focuses on the role of each health professional in the health care delivery system. The student has the opportunity to understand the preparation, emphasis, and responsibilities of other health professionals, to view his or her own profession within the context of the total health care system, and to explore strategies for expanding and improving interdisciplinary cooperation.

There is a close relationship between theory and process courses during these three semesters. The focus of the theory course determines the situation(s) within which the learnings in the process course will be utilized. For example, in the senior year the loss of patency unit addresses interrupted integrity in the cardiovascular system and obstruction in the gastrointestinal system. Students are expected to select clients in the clinical laboratory experiencing these hazardous events. (Laboratory activities will be discussed in greater detail in a later chapter.) Both theory and process courses are used to determine essential clinical experiences for all students.

Having completed the study of all stages of crisis and the nursing process, the student progresses to the eighth and final semester. This is a synthesis semester, and eight credits are allotted to the process course, "A Synthesis of Theory and Practice in Nursing." Clinical settings are categorized as pre-crisis, crisis, and post-crisis, and students are able to obtain an in-depth experience in an area of their choice. Classroom instruction concentrates on concepts related to management, consumer's rights, and change. There have been problems related to this course in terms of the exact content to be taught. In the early years of implementation there were annual changes and wide variations in content and techniques of classroom instruction, perhaps because the conceptual framework had not been clearly defined for this course. Another factor is that, for both faculty and students, the major investment is in the clinical component.

The theory course, "Nursing Practice—Today and Tomorrow," is a seminar course in which students consider broad philosophical issues that affect health needs and health care. Issues selected are those believed to have personal impact and, therefore, have the potential of conflict or crisis in one's professional practice. Topics are preselected by faculty and are reconsidered each year in order that they remain relevant to current issues.

5

Planning for Implementation
Jane Murdock

As curriculum planning progressed, it became increasingly clear that major organizational changes had to be initiated to facilitate the implementation of the new design. First, additional resources were essential to support the planned innovations. Second, programs had to be developed to orient students, faculty, and the staff of participating clinical agencies to their respective responsibilities. Finally, the faculty needed to be reorganized to adapt to an integrated curriculum. This chapter describes the actions taken in each of these three areas.

RESOURCES

Long-term planning was the key to securing the necessary resources for implementing the new curriculum. As early as 1970, two years prior to the entry of the first class into the revised lower division and four years prior to the first offering of the revised nursing major, the goals and the timetable for curriculum development were well established and incorporated into a five-year curriculum development project grant which was submitted to the Division of Nursing,

This chapter is adapted in part from Murdock, Jane. Regrouping for an Integrated Curriculum. Nursing Outlook (August 1978), Volume 26, No. 8. © American Journal of Nursing Co. Reproduced with permission.

Department of Health, Education, and Welfare in January 1971. Consequently, sufficient lead time was available to project needs and to acquire the necessary resources. Two categories of need were identified—physical facilities and personnel.

Physical Facilities

Space. Prior to initiating the new curriculum, the School of Nursing had only seven offices and one classroom in a small building on the university campus—all that was required since most of the activity of the school was then based within cooperating clinical agencies some distance from the main campus. Most faculty were housed in rented office space within the agencies, and almost all of the upper division nursing classes and conferences were held at these off-campus locations. With the new curriculum's emphasis on individualized, self-directed learning, and the fact that all four years of the program were to be campus-based, the acquisition of additional space on campus for offices, conference rooms, and a college laboratory was an urgent priority.

Through the committed efforts of the dean and the cooperation of the university administration, sufficient space to meet the immediate needs for offices and conference rooms was secured. Additional space was reserved for the college laboratory. After two years of intensive planning and major renovations, this long-awaited facility became a reality.

College Laboratory. The use of a college laboratory as an intermediary step between the classroom and the clinical laboratory was a major innovation of the new curricular approach. It was envisioned that the college laboratory, with its multimedia and simulated clinical divisions, would provide a setting in which students could acquire psychomotor skills, safely make errors, and become self-correcting and self-directed in their learning. In this setting, students could benefit not only from the individualized self-paced orientation of the media technology, but also from the opportunity to learn clinical skills apart from the demands of the real-life situation (University of Connecticut School of Nursing, 1977). The timely completion of the laboratory was essential to implementation of the new curriculum design.

Designing and equipping the laboratory was an enormous undertaking. Unfortunately, the magnitude of the task had not been fully appreciated prior to submitting the grant proposal. Although the need for funding for renovations and equipment had been anticipated and was available through the grant, no provision had been made for a staff position to oversee the planning and development of this facility. Recognizing the important of this task, the school's administration assigned a faculty member with expertise in multimedia instruction to devote 75 percent of her time to this endeavor. Without such an individual, implementation of the curriculum would have been seriously hampered.

Many activities had to be initiated simultaneously as the planning for the laboratory commenced. First, the advice of consultants was sought, and visits to college laboratories at other schools were planned. The information gained from these sources, in addition to a review of the literature and attendance at national meetings on multimedia instruction, was invaluable in finalizing the overall design of the laboratory and in suggesting guidelines for its operation.

Second, both the multimedia and simulated clinical divisions of the laboratory had to be equipped. After an extensive search of catalogues and other sources describing commercially available autotutorial programs, a variety of films, filmstrips, slides and audio and video tapes were ordered for faculty review and evaluation. A special evaluation form was prepared for this purpose. These evaluations were filed and used later when final media selections were made.

A similar search was undertaken to find appropriate equipment for both the media and the simulation laboratories. Factors such as cost, durability, ease of use, and repair were of major significance in all purchase decisions. The compatibility of the auto-tutorial equipment with the standard packaging of the commercially produced programs was of particular concern in selecting the equipment for the media laboratory.

Not only the type but also the amount of equipment to be purchased needed careful consideration. This was dependent upon the projected number of students and the amount of laboratory time needed per student. Just as important as the amount of time needed for viewing was the amount of space available to accommodate carrels and other equipment. Based on all the information that could be gathered, a decision was made to equip 20 individual study carrels, three group study areas, a large area for group viewing, and a storage and retrieval area.

In the simulated clinical laboratory, the estimated need included at least five fully equipped patient units, one treatment area, one medication area, space for both the storage and retrieval of equipment, and provision for viewing media and practicing skills simultaneously. All of the estimates were based on a projected enrollment of 160 students per class, with the laboratory operating on library hours. However, despite careful planning and a smaller enrollment than originally anticipated, it now appears that the laboratory is too small to meet the demands placed on it.

Another factor contributing to the effectiveness of any Instructional Media Laboratory is staffing. During the six years that this laboratory has been in operation, several different patterns have been utilized. There has always been a faculty member with media expertise in charge of that section of the laboratory, and two registered nurses with a minimum of a bachelor's degree in nursing in the simulated laboratory. Additional part-time support has been provided by graduate and undergraduate students (the latter in the media section only) and by faculty. The degree of responsibility of faculty for this aspect of the curriculum remains an unresolved issue.

Personnel

Faculty turnover was another problem associated with curriculum revision. As the time of implementation neared, the attrition rate accelerated rapidly. Almost a quarter of the faculty resigned during the two-year period immediately preceding the implementation of the revised nursing major. Many who left did so because they could not live comfortably with the anticipated changes. Appropriate replacements had to be hired and oriented quickly so that they could assume their responsibilities in both planning and implementation. Recruitment efforts were directed toward securing faculty who would be comfortable in a generalist role and have the type of clinical expertise needed to complement the skills of the faculty who had remained.

As prospective candidates were interviewed, considerable time was spent describing the curriculum and eliciting the applicant's reactions to it. Questions were asked such as: "How do you feel about an integrated curriculum? How comfortable would you be working with students outside your area of clinical expertise? Are you willing to learn to do this in at least one area other than your clinical specialty? How would you integrate the concepts from your specialty into a nursing component with a crisis theory framework?" In addition, each candidate had an opportunity to review the curriculum materials that had been developed. As a result, both the school and the applicant had a chance to make well-informed decisions. The interviewing team had an opportunity to evaluate the candidates and they, in turn, had a chance to decide if they wished to join the faculty.

FACULTY ORGANIZATION

Another problem in planning for implementation of the new curricular design was how to organize the faculty. It was obvious that the previous pattern of specialty teams was inappropriate for implementation of an integrated curriculum. However, the expertise of specialists was needed at each level of the program if we were to achieve both the classroom and clinical objectives. Two organizational changes were initiated to resolve this dilemma: faculty were organized into junior and senior level teams and, within each level, were assigned to clinical groups by geographic region.

Level Teams

Faculty with diverse clinical backgrounds were organized into two teams. One team was assigned responsibility for the courses of the junior level of the curriculum; the other team was assigned similar responsibility at the senior level. This seemed an appropriate way to assure the diversity of perspectives needed for the presentation of the new integrated courses. Although there were feelings about the loss of previous alliances and concerns about establishing new group relationships within this new pattern of organization, the faculty were relatively comfortable with this manner of organization.

Faculty preference for assignment to one of the level teams was ascertained through individual questionnaires and interviews. The final assignment was based on their preferences and the need for an equitable mix of specialty preparation within each level team. Most faculty were satisfied that these assignments were fair and that individual needs had been considered. Although the size of each team has varied yearly in relation to the size of the student population, the teams usually consist of 13 to 14 members.

Recognizing that trust in a leader is prerequisite to developing team relationships, the process of selecting a coordinator for each team was given careful consideration. The original plan of recruiting coordinators from outside the university was discarded in favor of selecting individuals who had participated in the curriculum's development and had demonstrated commitment to it as well as ability to work well with faculty colleagues. With these considerations in mind, each team was asked to submit the names of three faculty candidates to the dean who made the final appointments based on their recommendations. The appointments were for two years and were subject to review and renegotiation at the end of that time. The coordinators were charged with the overall responsibility for (1) the development, implementation and evaluation of courses at the respective level; (2) faculty orientation, development and evaluation; and (3) coordination between the two levels with the associate dean.

The teams agreed from the beginning that all major decisions affecting either level would be made by the total level team, and that all decisions affecting the total program would be made by the total undergraduate faculty. Within each level, task groups were organized to develop identified segments of courses, or deal with specific issues, and make recommendations to the level team for discussion and ratification. Membership of these groups was determined by the tasks to be accomplished. At times it was essential that each clinical specialty area be represented; at other times, a different criterion for selection was used. The outcome was that each faculty member came in contact with many other faculty and began to recognize previously unidentified strengths in her colleagues. Trust began to develop.

The coordinators served a vital role in identifying tasks to be accomplished, developing timetables, determining the need for specific groups, and facilitating the decision-making process by the total group. Both of the levels teams discovered that meetings were most productive when very specific proposals were presented to the group. These proposals, prepared either by task groups or the coordinator, served to focus the discussion and to facilitate the decision-making process.

Certain issues, such as the philosophy underlying the laboratory experience, program evaluation, and the objectives of the physical assessment component, had implications for both levels and were addressed in joint meetings of the two teams. Again, task groups were formed, this time composed of interlevel members. Recommendations were made by the task groups and discussed and ratified at interlevel meetings. This strategy increased faculty communication between levels and assured a unified approach to these dimensions of the curriculum. This large team pattern of organization can create problems, however—these are discussed in Chapter 8.

Clinical Regions

The implementation of a new curriculum design also affected the selection of clinical settings and the utilization of faculty. Previous territorial boundaries governing distribution of clinical resources were erased. As a preliminary step in redistribution, a survey was conducted of all resources within a 30-mile radius of campus. Many new agencies were identified and visited. Agencies previously utilized were reevaluated in terms of the new curriculum's requirements. Among the agencies surveyed were acute care centers, extended care facilities, schools, and physicians' offices. Data reflecting the philosophy and goals, geographic location, clientele, census statistics, staffing patterns, support services, and physical facilities of each agency were compiled and potential learning experiences within each agency were identified. This information was filed for future use.

Next, agencies were categorized and each category assigned a color code. A large map of the state was mounted on a cork board, and, using pins of corresponding colors, all agencies were charted on this map. It became apparent that the area was rich in resources. However, a system for distributing the wealth was needed, a system congruent with the demands of an integrated curriculum.

Since the new curriculum design prescribed a generalist, rather than specialist, role for faculty in meeting the clinical objectives related to crisis theory and nursing process, it was anticipated that students would be assigned to a faculty member rather than to an agency, and that students and faculty would function in a variety of settings in order to accomplish these objectives. Students were to assume an active role in the educational process. All activities were to be objective-centered, designed to enhance the students' problem-solving abilities and to encourage self-direction. Faculty were to provide guidance to support optimum learning and assist students in evaluating progress toward achieving learning goals.

Implementation of the clinical laboratory was the most emotionally charged issue of the entire process. Although the faculty tended to react as specialists, most believed the generalist approach to be valid and were committed to its pursuit. A new world of clinical teaching was opening up for most faculty—there were many unknowns. How, for example, would psychiatric and medical-surgical specialists function in each other's settings? Faculty were concerned about how they would function and where. An organizational pattern was thus needed to redraw territorial boundaries and to provide peer support for faculty in fulfilling the generalist role. The solution was the formation of clinical regions.

Clinical regions have geographic boundaries within which students and faculty seek resources to meet clinical objectives. A group of students, along with a team of faculty representative of the traditional specialty areas, is assigned to each region. Each faculty member acts as a preceptor for ten students and together the team plans the clinical learning activities for all students assigned to the region.

The regional boundaries were drawn on the survey map utilizing specific criteria. Since students at the junior level move frequently between the simulated setting of the college laboratory and the real setting of the clinical laboratory, proximity to the campus was an important consideration in establishing regional lines at this level. With senior students, the laboratory emphasis shifts to the clinical setting; college laboratory activities decrease markedly at this level and proximity is not as significant a factor. A more important consideration for the senior level was that of assuring availability of crisis-focused experiences in sufficient numbers to support a large student population. Since the campus is about 30 miles from a large metropolitan area, the lines for the senior regions were drawn to include this urban center where the concentrated client population provides an abundance of clinical resources. In all instances, the regional lines were drawn to assure an appropriate mix of clinical settings to support the focus of clinical objectives. The size of the regions, in terms of both geography and number of students, varied according to the resources available.

Students at each level are given the opportunity to state a preference for regional assignment; as might be suspected, some regions have been oversubscribed while others are undersubscribed. Faculty cannot fulfill all requests but try to minimize the travel difficulties and forestall the grievances that more arbitrary methods might have generated. A factor that is considered in addition to student preference is the importance of providing each student with a two-year clinical program that includes both urban and rural experiences. The availability of such varied experiences is a strength of the University of Connecticut curriculum.

Regional boundaries have been adjusted periodically on the basis of reassessment of resources and the learning needs of the assigned student population. Some regions have been decreased in size, others expanded. The concept remains intact and has been a useful strategy in implementing the clinical component. It has maximized the use of available resources and has provided faculty with a peer support system, thereby decreasing the threat and increasing the effectiveness of the generalist role.

ORIENTATION PROGRAMS

One key to the success of any new program is securing the support of the various groups affected by the change. In the case of the adoption of a new curriculum, the people most intimately affected are the faculty who are expected to implement it and the students who will experience it. Another group that is important to the success of a nursing curriculum is the staff of the agencies that provide clinical experiences. Provisions for orientation of these three interest groups was an integral part of curriculum planning.

Faculty

When candidates were interviewed they were given sufficient information about the new curriculum to help them decide if they wished to join the faculty. A crucial time for the new faculty member and for the new curriculum proved to be the first year of employment. It was recognized that the newcomers should have input into planning and decision-making, but the faculty was determined that issues which had been already resolved should not be called into question all over again, and that decisions already made should not be reopened before they had been adequately tested. Otherwise deadlines would slip by and students would be subjected to a hastily conceived, superficially developed program.

An orientation program was designed to help new faculty understand the decision-making process, including some of the ideas that had been proposed and discarded, so they would be supportive of the new design and not seek drastic changes until it had been carefully evaluated.

A valuable resource for orientation was the annual curriculum project reports. These reports, along with two unpublished papers on crisis theory written by two faculty members, were given to all newcomers during the early years of implementation. A series of orientation meetings was sponsored by the curriculum project committee as an aid to understanding and internalizing the reports. These meetings examined in depth the various components of the curriculum and the process by which they were developed. Topics included lower division and upper division courses, the theoretical framework, the advisement system, philosophy of laboratory, and the evaluation model.

As the curriculum became firmly established, the task of orienting new faculty members to it was assumed by the level coordinators: other aspects of orientation became the responsibility of the Faculty Affairs Committee. A brief history of the curriculum eventually became part of the faculty handbook given to all faculty along with updated curriculum materials. And this book may itself probably become required reading for all new faculty.

Students

Prior to admission of the first class to the revised curriculum, an advisement system was established. Under this system, each entering student is assigned a school of nursing faculty advisor who provides academic counseling throughout the four-year program. The advisor initially explains the various course requirements, explores any special needs or interests with the student, and individualizes the program as much as possible within the prescribed limits.

This student/faculty advisor relationship is especially important because the curriculum does not include any nursing courses during the first year. The advisement system is a mechanism for keeping beginning students in touch with the school of nursing and providing them with a person who can respond to their questions and concerns about the program and about nursing. The faculty advisor also monitors the students' progress and assists in the registration process so that lower division requirements are met on schedule.

Two advisement manuals were also developed, one for students and one for faculty advisors. These manuals explain the advisement system, the mechanics of the registration process, the rationale for the lower division courses, and alternatives to facilitate individualization of the program. The student manual was revised in 1978 to include a description of the nursing component in greater detail and to answer questions most frequently asked by students. This manual is now given to prospective students as well as incoming ones during the summer orientation period.

During the early years of implementation of the integrated curriculum, the advisement system and manuals assisted in the orientation of students but they were not enough. Because the program was new and had no graduates or even upper division students to describe their experiences, many class meetings were needed to deal with the rumors, answer questions, and provide reassurance. With the curriculum firmly established, the frequency of meetings diminished but an annual or semi-annual meeting for each class continues to be an important means of disseminating information and keeping in touch with student concerns.

Agency Staff

The new curriculum design and the newly-designated clinical regions meant marked changes in the role of agencies utilized for clinical experiences; the support and cooperation of agency staff would be essential to effective implementation of such changes. The key to securing this support was in providing information and promulgating the new ideas so that agency personnel would be willing to participate in the program.

A series of day-long orientation programs for agency staff was instituted. The initial one took place nine months before the first class entered the new clinical courses. The programs included the reason for curriculum revisions, the goals of the new plan, an overview of the conceptual framework, and a description of the nursing courses.

An attempt was made to present the material in a way that would be meaningful to service personnel and convince them that faculty were trying to prepare practitioners to meet their needs. Guidelines for the use of the clinical laboratory were distributed and discussed at length. Questions were answered and concerns responded to, many of which reflected age-old criticisms of baccalaureate education. The orientation programs were not completely successful in dispelling doubts and securing cooperation, although they did represent a first step in a continuing public relations campaign.

Several factors contributed to the differences in the nature of the newly-designed clinical activities and the need to prepare agencies for these differences. First, clinical activities were to be selected to meet objectives derived from the crisis model and appropriate to a specific step in the nursing process. Also, students would be using crisis theory language to discuss their clients. Second, because of the integrated curriculum, faculty were to function as generalists and students were to be assigned to faculty rather than to agencies. Third, the newly-developed philosophy of laboratory was expected to markedly influence the selection of learning activities, the nature of faculty guidance, and the relationship between agency staff, faculty, and students. These factors are discussed in detail in Chapter 7 and some associated problems are described in Chapter 8.

A fourth change was in the greater number and variety of agencies that had been explored as potential sources of student experience—some of these had never had students before. Faculty were not sure if it would be more difficult for new agencies to accept the innovative program or for previously used agencies to adapt to it. Invitations to the orientation programs were extended to personnel of all the agencies that had indicated an interest in having students. No commitment was expected from them at that time.

It was decided that several faculty members and two, or even three, levels of students might use a given agency at various times during a semester. In order to provide for the coordination of activities and to foster good relationships between school and agency, a liaison system was established. Under this system one faculty member is appointed as a liaison for each agency. All arrangements for clinical experiences are to be initially channeled through that individual. The following responsibilities were developed for the liaison faculty member.

1. Facilitate communication between the agency and the university faculty and administration.
2. Communicate to faculty the potential availability of learnings.
3. Interpret to the agency the purposes and goals of the school.
4. Discuss with the agency personnel the learning needs of students. When two levels of students are utilizing an agency, this responsibility will be shared by the representatives from each level.
5. Keep the agency informed of names of faculty and students using the agency.
6. Be of assistance to the agency by providing consultation, assisting with inservice programs, etc.
7. Provide the agency with feedback in relation to student experiences.
8. Arrange with the agency for end of year evaluation conference.
9. Write a thank you letter at the end of the year.
10. Update the agency file in the School of Nursing.

This system has proved to be an effective means of monitoring the flow of traffic, strengthening relationships with agency personnel, and clarifying the aims of the curriculum.

6

Course Development

Edna Johnson
Linda R. Suess
Marguerite B. White

In May 1974, the junior level faculty faced the formidable task of translating the conceptual framework, course descriptions, and the grid into fully developed fifth semester courses—courses complete with objectives, units of content, teaching strategies, study guides, and evaluative techniques. Although the objectives for the junior level had been developed, both classroom and clinical learning experiences appropriate to the objectives needed to be identified including selection of software for the media laboratory, activities for the simulated and clinical laboratories, and clinical agencies appropriate for the newly-designed objectives.

To accomplish the task, the faculty divided into two groups, one for each course, during the summer of 1974. The essential tasks were completed by the first of September. The remaining tasks became part of the ongoing activities for the academic year and were accomplished through weekly meetings of the total team, supplemented by work in small groups.

In planning for sixth semester courses, a different strategy was used in order to facilitate correlation of theory with process. Several task groups were formed, and each group was assigned two loss categories. In addition to developing content, objectives, study guides, and bibliographies for the theory course, each group developed the corresponding unit in the process course. The correlation between sixth semester theory and process courses can be seen in figure 6-3. Weekly meetings were held, and the level coordinator was kept informed of progress and problems. By the beginning of the spring semester, the course outlines were ready and teaching responsibilities had been allocated.

Senior year faculty had an entire year in which to develop the courses that they would be teaching beginning in September 1975. This proved to be a mixed blessing. They had to deal with the problems associated with teaching seniors in the outgoing curriculum concurrent with planning for seniors in the new one. Some of these problems are described in Chapter 8.

The remainder of this chapter presents some of the outcomes of this period in the curriculum development process. The first section illustrates the objectives for a three semester sequence of nursing courses, the second examines the content for one strand, and the third traces the development of content relating to one of the major concepts through a three semester sequence. Lastly, the synthesis semester is briefly described, the crisis theory approach to nursing content is summarized, and its advantages are identified.

LEVELS OF OBJECTIVES
CRISIS THEORY/PROCESS

An objective is a statement of what the student is expected to do upon completion of a particular learning segment. Program objectives are developed in a very early stage of curriculum development and are appropriately global in nature. Course objectives need to be congruent with these program objectives but must also describe behaviors that are measurable and attainable in a time period of one semester.

The crisis theory formulation provided the major concepts to be included in the objectives for the junior and senior level courses. (These concepts are described in Chapter 3.) More precise guidance for individual course objectives was obtained from course descriptions and the grid. Selected objectives from upper division nursing courses are presented in figures 6-1 and 6-2.

The progression of learning is reflected in these objectives. The movement is from developmental hazardous events to situational, then to combined situational and developmental events; from pre-crisis to crisis to post-crisis; and from wellness to illness and then to the highest possible level of wellness. (The rationale for this sequence was explained in Chapter 4.) In comparing the objectives with the crisis model (figure 3-1), it is clear that each objective describes an activity the student must be able to perform in order to achieve the nursing goal for a stage of the crisis model. It should also be clear that these objectives are only samples, they are not all-inclusive. If all objectives from all nursing courses were presented, every element of the conceptual model would theoretically be identifiable.

First Level: Health/Assessment

Faculty charged with the development of the first level of clinical nursing content knew that the major concepts to be developed were wellness, developmental hazardous events, pre-crisis, and assessment. Therefore, content of the theory course had to include a study of representative hazardous events at each developmental stage, of wellness behaviors for the individual throughout the life span, and of interventions to achieve the nursing goals of the pre-crisis stage (health promotion and disease prevention through anticipatory guidance, augmentation of the person's coping mechanisms and/or reduction of the hazardous potential of specific events). The objectives for the first level, listed in figure 6-1, show some of the actions expected of the student in relation to these major concepts.

Concurrent with the study of nursing theory, students need to acquire the intellectual and psychomotor skills required to assess individuals and/or families and to prevent crisis. These activities are apparent in the objectives of the first level process course (figure 6-2). The focus of the theory course determines the situation in which the learnings of the process course will be applied. Therefore, the process course objectives not only address the various steps in assessment, but also provide direction for the assessment and are consistent with the wellness component of the health-illness continuum. Prevention of crisis, a nursing goal in the pre-crisis stage, is apparent in the objectives of both courses at this level. Developmental hazardous events, which are the simplest to deal with because they are predictable, are identified.

Second Level: Illness/Planning and Intervention

The objectives of the second level courses illustrate the second step in the sequence. Since the focus is on illness and situational hazardous events, which have less predictability than developmental ones, the theory course objectives listed in figure 6-1 reflect these concepts and are consistent with the second stage of the crisis model when the

Theory Course, Level 1 (Nursing 203)

Outlines the components of one or more developmental hazardous events which occur at each stage on the developmental continuum.

Selects from given descriptions of behaviors those indicative of imminent psychosocial and/or psychological crisis in response to developmental hazardous events.

Gives several examples of coping mechanisms used to reduce anxiety and to avert crisis.

Utilizes health concepts to assess the individual's/family's levels of wellness.

Theory Course, Level 2 (Nursing 223)

Outlines the components of one or more situational hazardous events occurring in each loss category.

Describes the effect on the individual/family of selected situational hazardous events in each loss category.

Gives examples of problem solving mechanisms used to resolve problems resulting from situational hazardous events.

Describes additional internal and external resources used to resolve problems when the individual/family is in crisis.

Theory Course, Level 3 (Nursing 233)

Recognizes the combination(s) of situational and developmental hazards which place a client at risk for crisis.

Recognizes bio-psycho-social behaviors of the client in crisis.

Discriminates between those internal/external resources that may or may not be mobilized for or by the client.

Describes the possible avenues of crisis resolution.

Distinguishes between those immediate interventions necessary to minimize disorganization in crisis and those additional interventions leading to bio-psycho-social growth.

Recognizes interventions which assist the client to move from maladaptive behavior(s) toward those behaviors indicative of his maximum level of wellness.

FIGURE 6-1. Selected theory course objectives illustrating levels of learning.

Process Course, Level 1 (Nursing 208)

1.0 Assesses the level of health of the individual/family of varying ages who possess characteristics of wellness.
    1.1 Collects relevant data.
    1.5 Demonstrates use of tools and technics necessary to make a health examination.
    1.6 Records data collected.
    1.7 Analyzes and interprets collected data.

3.0 States a Nursing Diagnosis.
    3.1 Identifies existing and potential problems of individual/family.
    3.2 Identifies existing and potential strengths of individual/family.
    3.4 Describes mechanisms used by individual/family for coping.
    3.5 Identifies resources utilized by individual/family.

Process Course, Level 2 (Nursing 228)

2.0 Designs a plan of nursing care based on assessment of individuals/families in various stages of crisis resulting from situational or developmental hazardous events.
    2.1 Assesses selected individuals/families for losses in the following categories: relationships, mobility, regulation, patency, protective mechanisms, and sensory-motor exchange.
    2.2 Determines priorities for resolution of problems identified in the assessment process.

3.0 Implements the plan.
    3.1 Utilizes psychomotor skills accurately and safely.
    3.2 Utilizes interpersonal skills in an appropriate manner.

Process Course, Level 3 (Nursing 238)

1.0 Assesses individuals and/or families in stages of crisis resulting from combinations of developmental and situational hazardous events.
    1.1 Identifies intrinsic and extrinsic factors which influence growth, maintenance, and/or maladaptation.
    1.2 Predicts the possible avenues of crisis resolution.

2.0 Designs a plan for intervention which mobilizes existing and additional resources.
    2.4 Identifies methods of evaluation appropriate to planned intervention(s).

3.0 Implements, in collaboration with the health team, the plan of nursing intervention for clients in stages of crisis.

4.0 Evaluates the client's behavioral response to the intervention(s).

5.0 Evaluates self-growth.

FIGURE 6-2. Selected process course objectives illustrating levels of learning.

nursing goal is amelioration or cure through mobilization of additional resources. The planning and intervention steps in the nursing process are apparent in the objectives of the process course (figure 6-2).

Third Level: Complex Situations/Evaluation

The third level nursing courses deal with more complex illness situations in which the client is at greater risk for crisis and with post-crisis resolution. The final phase of the nursing process—evaluation—is emphasized. There are two major objectives relating to evaluation, one referring to client behavior and the other to the practitioner's behavior. At this third level, the illness back to wellness part of the sequence and the goals of nursing interventions in the post-crisis phase, which are rehabilitation and/or maintenance, are evident in the objectives of both courses. All the steps in the nursing process, with special emphasis on evaluation, are utilized for clients in various stages of crisis resulting from a combination of developmental and situational hazardous events.

In summary, the concept of simple-to-complex is seen in the sequence of course objectives. The progression from the predictable developmental hazardous events to the combined developmental-situational hazardous events, which are least predictable, is illustrated. The location on the health-illness continuum and the stage of crisis are made clear in the objectives of each theory course. One step of the nursing process is added to the previous step(s) in the process course objectives.

The wording of the objectives listed in figures 6-1 and 6-2 is not completely consistent among the levels. They all utilize the conceptual framework accurately but the variations in expression are reflective of differences in writing style. This is a problem to be expected when curriculum materials are being developed simultaneously by different groups of faculty. Perhaps a next step would be rewording of the objectives for all courses by representatives from both junior and senior levels.

If complete objectives for the six courses described above are reviewed carefully, all of the concepts from the crisis model become apparent. In addition, there are objectives relating to each of the strands in which levels of learning can be clearly identified. As courses were developed, the strands were incorporated into the theory/process content. The health teaching strand offers an interesting illustration.

HEALTH TEACHING STRAND

First Level: Health/Assessment

The first level process course emphasizes assessment in levels of health. On the grid, the health teaching content for this course is identified as follows: maintenance of health—primary prevention; identification of learning needs; assessment of learner; principles of teaching; principles of learning; development of plan for teaching; implementation of plan; revision of plan as necessary. Learning experiences to achieve the health teaching objective include readings, class hours, and a health teaching project.

The project requires each student to select a client and identify a learning need related to health promotion for example, self breast examination for a female client or proper dental care for a preschooler. Having identified the need, the student assesses the learner, then develops and implements a teaching plan. The written report of the project, which comprises twenty percent of the course grade, includes the detailed teaching plan, the principles of learning that were illustrated, and a brief assessment of the effectiveness of the teaching. In other words, were the objectives met? In what ways was the plan good? In what ways could it have been improved?

In addition to the above project, students participate in a variety of clinical experiences where they may observe the health teaching activities of other professionals or have an opportunity to engage in health teaching themselves. For example, a student may observe prenatal or planned parenthood classes and/or participate in health teaching activities related to the needs of the postpartum client, the newborn, and its father.

Since the first level theory course focuses on primary prevention and pre-crisis, and the outcome of developmental hazardous events can be influenced by health teaching, this is a major nursing intervention in the pre-crisis stage. For example, teaching expectant parents about labor and delivery is thought to lessen the probability of a crisis. As the first level courses were being developed, faculty debated the appropriateness of including teaching, which is an intervention, in a course that focuses on assessment. A purist might say it was inappropriate, but the faculty decided that it was logical for students to learn and apply the principles of teaching when they are focusing on well clients. A study of pre-crisis would be incomplete if assessment of the level of health and determination of health teaching needs were not followed by interventions appropriate to achieve the nursing

goal of that crisis stage. Teaching is, without doubt, an integral
part of health maintenance and promotion. This is an example of a
curriculum decision that was guided by the conceptual framework.

Second Level: Illness/Planning and Intervention

Since the second level process course deals with individuals and/or
families who are experiencing situational hazardous events which
may precipitate a crisis, the emphasis in this semester is on health
teaching as it applies to the prevention or resolution of such events.
One example of a situational hazardous event is surgery. A clinical
activity expected of the student is assessment of a pre-surgical client
to identify learning needs as evidenced by his perception of the surgical intervention. The principles learned in the previous semester
are applied to this situation. A teaching plan based upon the client's
needs is developed and implemented. The student has an opportunity
to evaluate the outcomes of this teaching by observing and caring for
the client postoperatively.

In the accompanying theory course, problem-solving mechanisms used to resolve situational hazardous events are studied. One
of the nurse's activities in assisting an individual to resolve problems
related to situational hazardous events is health teaching. For example, the individual with loss of hormonal regulation that results in
diabetes is in need of specific instructions in order to modify his life
style and prevent further illness. This illustrates the application of
skills learned in the process course to the situations studied in the
theory course.

Third Level: Complex Situations/Evaluation

As identified on the grid, the content of the third level process course
includes: refinement of teaching skills; evaluation of learning or non-
learning; factors which interfere with learning; reinforcement of
learning; re-teaching; and group teaching. The individual experiencing
post-crisis adaptation to a changed level of wellness is a focus of the
theory course. An example is the client with abnormal respiratory
conditions. Clients with pulmonary obstructive disease have a chronic
illness which causes a permanent impairment of respiration and requires changes in life style to function effectively. Therefore, health
teaching tends to be more complex than for a client experiencing a

short-term hazardous event such as surgery where the outcome is expected to be complete recovery.

Since the focus of the course is on the evaluation component of the nursing process, it is appropriate to emphasize the evaluation of health teaching activities. Strategies are developed to effect change in behavior when initial health teaching has not been successful. In addition, students become involved in group teaching and apply principles of learning and of evaluation to that situation.

CONCEPT OF MOBILITY

To illustrate the utilization of the crisis model, as well as the simple to complex sequence and the correlation between theory and process courses, the concept of mobility will be traced through the three semester sequence. Mobility is defined as "the potential to move from one area to another, physically, socially, and/or psychologically." The sections of the grid that provided direction for developing this content area are reproduced in figure 6-3.

First Level: Health/Assessment

In the first level clinical nursing course, content is organized around developmental tasks or changes. The only item on the grid under "mobility" is "accidents." Instead of treating this content as a separate unit, it is subsumed within the unit entitled "Adaptation to Change in Physical Status." The close relationship between an individual's physical status and his level of mobility supports this placement of content. While all age levels are included in this unit, infants, children, and the elderly are emphasized because of particular hazards present at these times—achieving an increasing level of mobility in a child and coping with a decreasing level in the elderly.

In the theory course, content for this unit begins with identification of the hazardous events associated with changes in mobility. One such event in early childhood is learning to crawl. This event occurs when the neurological system of the child matures through the process of myelinization. Since cognitive development does not keep pace with physical development, the child learns this motor skill—crawling—before he learns to make judgments about how to use this skill safely. Therefore, myelinization coupled with lag in cognitive development is an intrinsic factor that places the child at risk.

Semester 5	Semester 6	Semester 7
Theory NURS 203	Theory NURS 223	Theory NURS 233
Adaptation to Change in Physical Status	Loss of Mobility	Loss of Mobility
Nutrition	Physical Immobility	Psychological Immobility
Elimination	Bedrest	Specific Hazardous Events:
Sensory Acuity	Loss of Function	Chronicity
Hormonal Levels	Psychological Immobility	Early Onset
Level of Wellness	Isolation	Late Onset
Mobility	Specific Hazardous Events:	Loss of Sensory-Motor Exchanges
Accidents	Cerebral Vascular Accident	Destruction of Nervous System
	Fractures	Degeneration
Process	Congenital Hip	Trauma
NURS 208	Amputation	Distortion
	Gifted/Retarded Individual	Inflammation
Intellectual Skills		Pressure
Assessment of Individual/Family	Process	Specific Hazardous Events:
Observation	NURS 228	Head Injury
Wellness Baseline		Spinal Cord Injury
Data Base	Psychomotor Skills	Meningitis
Collection	Loss of Mobility	Meningomyelocele
Analysis	Comfort and Hygiene	Multiple Sclerosis
Interpretation	Bedbath	
Validation	Bedmaking	
Health History	Backrub	
Problem/Strength Lists	Specialized Skin Care	
Recording	Body Mechanics	
Subjective Data	Exercise Regimens	
Objective Data	Positioning and Protective Devices	
Psychomotor Skills	Assistive Devices	
Physical Assessment	Ambulation Techniques	
	Cast Care	
	Binders and Splints	
	Prostheses	
	Traction	
	Diversional Activities	
	Specific Hazardous Events:	
	Spica Cast, Fractured Leg	

FIGURE 6–3. Mobility and loss of mobility (excerpt from grid).

External risk factors also may be present. For example, a parent beset with personal problems and careless about a child's welfare, or a room with an unprotected staircase, place the child at risk for injury when he begins to crawl. On the other hand, an overprotective environment is a risk factor because it may delay achievement of mobility.

Another influencing factor is the parents' perception of the event. If the parents are proud of the child's accomplishment and pleased at this sign of normal development, the child will also be proud and happy and will become increasingly mobile. If the parents are anxious, on the other hand, the child may become frightened and decrease rather than increase his mobility. Parents who expect too much and push a child to be mobile before he is ready may also adversely affect the accomplishment of this developmental task.

Nursing actions during this stage include assessment, anticipatory guidance, and health teaching to achieve the goals of health promotion and disease (accident) prevention. In the process course, students acquire the skills of interviewing, history taking, and physical assessment, including the administration of the Denver Developmental Screening Test. These tools are needed to collect data upon which to base the plan for nursing interventions. Such data include information about the child's fine and gross motor skills, his intellectual achievements, the hazards in his environment, and his parents' problem-solving mechanisms.

An example of a nursing intervention is helping the parents to perceive the event (learning to crawl) realistically, to know what to expect, to perceive the dangers in the situation, and to foster the child's growth by encouraging mobility. When parents perceive the dangers inherent in the event, they can be helped to think preventively in order to create a safe environment by such actions as placing a gate across an open stairway, adding safety latches to doors, or moving poisonous substances out of reach. The health teaching plan also includes the provision of any needed information about accident prevention, future mobility changes to be anticipated (learning to walk), sensory stimulation, nutrition, and appropriate toys and activities to stimulate the child mentally while enhancing his fine and gross motor skills.

Learning to crawl is but one example of a hazardous event associated with achieving mobility. In the fifth semester theory course, all such events occurring at each age level are identified and described, including the intrinsic and extrinisic factors associated with risk and the nursing interventions to prevent crisis. Developmental theory provides the base for this content. The process and techniques of assessment are taught in the accompanying process course. Related clinical laboratory experiences take place in schools, day-care centers, clinics, physicians' offices, and homes.

At the other end of the age continuum, the elderly are studied in relation to the concepts of mobility, health, and pre-crisis. In direct antithesis to the child's increasing mobility, the elderly must cope with the hazardous event of a declining level of mobility. As an individual ages, certain intrinsic factors place him at risk for injuries that could result in disability and hospitalization. For example, a decrease occurs in the size of the musculature as well as in the density of bone structure. There may be some reduction, also, in reaction time to stimulus. These changes may lead to a level of mobility reflective of decreased muscle strength, agility, and stamina.

The elderly are sensitive to any changes in their level of physical mobility since a decrease can signal the end of a valued independent life style. To surrender a driver's license or to sell one's home and move to a small apartment in an elderly housing complex can be very disturbing. These are extrinsic factors that produce a social as well as emotional impact and may contribute to a psychological immobility and increase the risk of crisis. Additionally, after retirement the circle of associates may be reduced in numbers, family and friends may die, and a decreased physical mobility may prohibit much interaction with others. The elderly need mental stimulation to remain alert and responsive to the environment.

The focus of nursing action to prevent crisis is assessment followed by appropriate health teaching. Assessment of mobility in the elderly includes both physiological and psychosocial factors. A thorough health history may identify past or current conditions that have potential for the development of mobility problems, for example, past injuries or illnesses, the presence of chronic diseases, or the intake of medications that may affect the sensorium and/or the neuromuscular systems. A history may also reveal changes in the individual's ability to perform his own activities of daily living.

Through physical assessment intrinsic factors that place the individual at risk may be discovered. For example, assessment of vision may show decreased acuity that could lead to accidents or injuries. Assessing the neuromuscular systems may detect diminishing muscle size or strength or neurologic deficits such as decreased reflexes or loss of peripheral sensations.

Assessment of the home is essential in order to identify any extrinsic factors that may cause an accident and lead to a decrease in mobility. Such factors might include loose rugs, electrical cords in walking areas, poor lighting, or absence of handrails on stairs. In the psychological realm, it is important to determine the individual's orientation and identify interaction patterns with others.

Included in health teaching for the elderly individual may be suggestions for protection from hazards in the home; for example, securing rugs, using a night light or a commode at night. The client can be taught to use shoes with non-skid soles, to use assistive devices (such as a cane or walker) when indicated, and to consume a diet supportive to his needs. The elderly individual can also be encouraged to take full advantage of available community resources that might enhance the level of mobility and overall health status. Such resources may include a senior center, Meals on Wheels, Dial A Ride, and the Visiting Nurse.

In order to apply content related to mobility at this age level, students have clinical experiences with the elderly in senior citizen centers, rest homes or nursing homes, and in the client's home. Activities include physical and psychosocial assessment followed by health teaching. If deviations from normal are noted, referral to the appropriate resource is initiated.

In summary, the first level courses examine the concept of mobility in relation to developmental changes. All phases of the life span are included but attention is focused on the periods when the risk is greatest—childhood and old age. Nursing activities are primarily assessment and health teaching which are appropriate for the pre-crisis stage of the crisis model. Knowledge gained during this semester is utilized in subsequent semesters when illness (crisis and post-crisis) and additional steps in the nursing process are examined.

Second Level: Illness/Planning and Intervention

The first level courses dealt with achievement of mobility and a natural decline in that function. In the second level courses, which are illness-oriented, loss of mobility is viewed as a situational hazardous event. The emphasis is on the crisis engendered or threatened by the loss

In the theory course, the mobility unit begins with generalizations: what hazardous events will cause a loss of mobility, either physical or psychological or both? How does the loss affect the individual and family? Emphasis is on the factors that are common results of disparate events, for example, as a result of a heart attack, a fractured bone, a cerebral vascular accident, or a catatonic state. Age-related concepts such as the impact of mobility on the developmental needs of the client are considered. The concept of isolation is introduced as an example of a psychological immobility.

After the students understand the generalizations about mobility, a variety of specific hazardous events are studied. Students learn to apply these new generalizations to concrete situations and continue to apply the health-related concepts as well as basic science principles from other courses. By studying a few representative events, they learn how to apply the crisis model and also acquire a body of knowledge to be used in the future with any client experiencing this loss.

The specific events chosen to illustrate loss of mobility are cerebrovascular accident, fractures, congenital hip, amputation, and the gifted/retarded individual. A study of these events encompasses many age levels and provides opportunity for students to utilize many basic nursing skills. Also, some of them are common health problems, often seen by students in the clinical setting. A brief sketch of some of the content relating to cerebrovascular accident will illustrate the use of the crisis model. This content is presented graphically in figures 6-4 - 6-9. The biophysical and psychosocial models are diagrammed separately for clarity.

Although the focus of the sixth semester is on intervening in crises resulting from situational hazardous events, discussion always begins with consideration of the pre-crisis stage. What are the factors that place the client at risk? In this case they are such elements as age, hypertension, family history, diet, lack of adequate health care. The nursing interventions in this stage (case finding, health teaching, and referral) are also discussed. Figure 6-4 presents the pre-crisis phase of the biophysical model.

In diagramming the psychosocial model (figure 6-5), discovery of hypertension might have been identified as the hazardous event that initiated the client's problem-solving mechanisms. Instead, the writer chose to diagram the events following the client's perception of mobility loss resulting from the cerebrovascular accident. This illustrates the point that crisis is not the event itself, but the response to the event. In this particular situation, intervention could not avert a biophysical crisis but it might avert a psychosocial one. Figure 6-5 lists the problem-solving mechanisms and the nursing actions that are initiated to avert a crisis.

When body defenses and/or coping mechanisms fail, crisis ensues—physical or psychosocial or both. Content at this stage centers on a description of the behaviors that are indicative of crisis; the additional resources that are mobilized; nursing actions to augment the coping mechanisms of the individual or family; and measures to prevent complications and achieve a positive resolution of

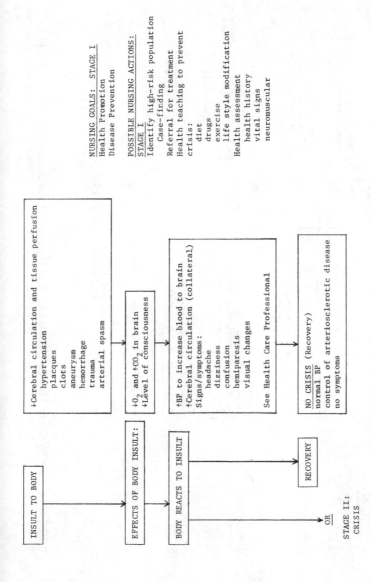

FIGURE 6-4. Biophysical model: loss of mobility (cerebrovascular accident). Stage I: Pre-crisis.

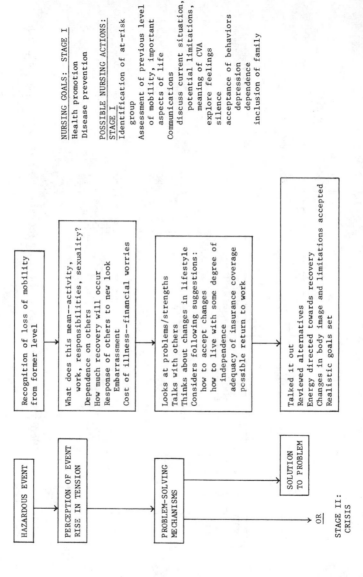

NURSING GOALS: STAGE I
Health promotion
Disease prevention

POSSIBLE NURSING ACTIONS:
STAGE I
Identification of at-risk
    group
Assessment of previous level
    of mobility, important
    aspects of life
Communications
discuss current situation,
    potential limitations,
    meaning of CVA
explore feelings
silence
acceptance of behaviors
    depression
    dependence
    inclusion of family

Recognition of loss of mobility
from former level

What does this mean—activity,
    work, responsibilities, sexuality?
Dependence on others
How much recovery will occur
Response of others to new look
Embarrassment
Cost of illness--financial worries

Looks at problems/strengths
Talks with others
Thinks about changes in lifestyle
Considers following suggestions:
    how to accept changes
    how to live with some degree of
        independence
    adequacy of insurance coverage
    possible return to work

Talked it out
Reviewed alternatives
Energy directed towards recovery
Changes in body image and limitations accepted
Realistic goals set

HAZARDOUS EVENT

PERCEPTION OF EVENT
RISE IN TENSION

PROBLEM-SOLVING
MECHANISMS

SOLUTION
TO PROBLEM

OR

STAGE II:
CRISIS

FIGURE 6-5. Psychosocial model: loss of mobility (cerebrovascular accident). Stage I:
Pre-crisis.

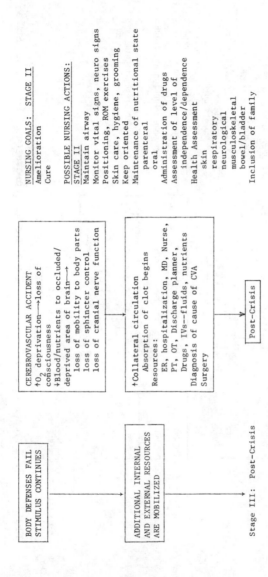

FIGURE 6-6. Biophysical model: Loss of mobility (cerebrovascular accident). Stage II: Crisis.

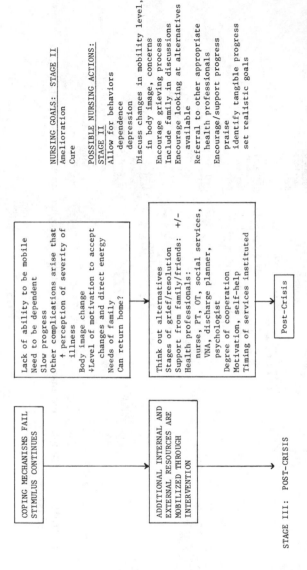

NURSING GOALS: STAGE II
Amelioration
Cure

POSSIBLE NURSING ACTIONS:
STAGE II
Allow for behaviors
  dependence
  depression
Discuss changes in mobility level,
  in body image, concerns
Encourage grieving process
Include family in discussions
Encourage looking at alternatives
  available
Referral to other appropriate
  health professionals
Encourage/support progress
  praise
  identify tangible progress
  set realistic goals

COPING MECHANISMS FAIL
STIMULUS CONTINUES

Lack of ability to be mobile
Need to be dependent
Slow progress
Other complications arise that
  ↑ perception of severity of
  illness
Body image change
↓Level of motivation to accept
  changes and direct energy
Needs of family
Can return home?

Think out alternatives
Stages of grief/resolution
Support from family/friends: +/-
Health professionals:
  nurse, PT, OT, social services,
  VNA, discharge planner,
  psychologist
Degree of cooperation
Motivation, self-help
Timing of services instituted

ADDITIONAL INTERNAL AND
EXTERNAL RESOURCES ARE
MOBILIZED THROUGH
INTERVENTION

Post-Crisis

STAGE III: POST-CRISIS

FIGURE 6-7. Psychosocial model: Loss of mobility (cerebrovascular accident). Stage II: Crisis.

102

the crisis. These include prevention of the hazards of immobility, measures to increase mobility, and assisting the client to accept limitations. Figures 6-6 and 6-7 diagram the crisis phase of this hazardous event.

The students' knowledge of assessment is augmented at this time to include recognition of such unhealthy responses to the event as skin breakdown, infection, and maladaptive behavior. Students are also expected to transfer knowledge of concepts taught in previous units to this individual with mobility loss. Such concepts include the sick role (loss of relationships), inflammation and pain (loss of protective mechanisms), and the many concepts subsumed in the surgical cycle (under loss of regulation).

Although examination of the post-crisis phase of the crisis model provides the focus for the seventh semester courses, the study of a situational hazardous event and resultant crisis would be incomplete without planning for recovery. Therefore, content related to the post-crisis phase of cerebrovascular accident is included. (See figures 6-8 and 6-9.)

Content in the sixth semester nursing process course complements the theory related to loss of mobility. Students discuss the planning and intervention needed in caring for an individual coping with such a loss. In addition, psychomotor skills related to loss of mobility are learned and utilized. Such skills include measures of comfort and hygiene, body mechanics, positioning, ambulation techniques, and diversional activities (see figure 6-3). Related clinical experiences take place in hospitals, extended care facilities, and the home.

To summarize, the second level courses introduce the concept of loss of mobility and focus primarily on the crisis stage of the model using several common health problems as examples. Concepts from previous courses related to health and assessment are applied to the ill individual, with the addition of the next steps in the nursing process-planning and intervention. Students apply these concepts to individuals coping with loss of mobility during clinical laboratory experiences in acute care, long term, and home environments.

Third Level—Complex Situations/Evaluation

The third level nursing courses focus on the final aspects of the crisis model and the nursing process—crisis/post-crisis and intervention/evaluation. In addition, previously learned concepts related to the health-illness continuum, the pre-crisis and crisis stages, and the initial steps of the nursing process are now applied to more

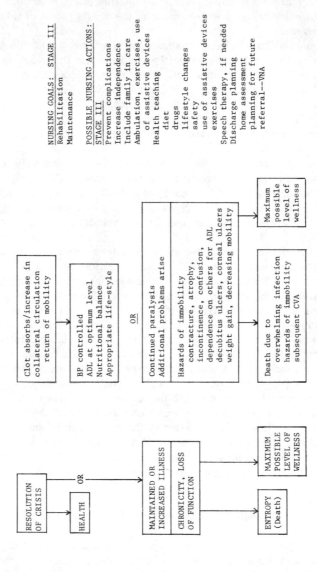

FIGURE 6-8. Biophysical model: loss of mobility (cerebrovascular accident). Stage III: Post-crisis.

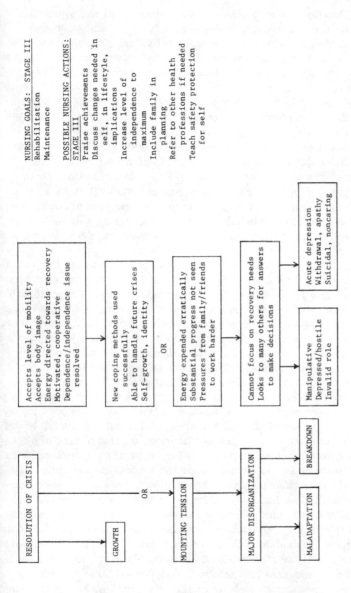

NURSING GOALS: STAGE III
Rehabilitation
Maintenance

POSSIBLE NURSING ACTIONS:
STAGE III
Praise achievements
Discuss changes needed in
    self, in lifestyle,
    implications
Increase level of
    independence to
    maximum
Include family in
    planning
Refer to other health
    professions if needed
Teach safety protection
    for self

FIGURE 6-9. Psychosocial model: loss of mobility (cerebrovascular accident). Stage III: Post-crisis.

105

complex situations. Crises with both developmental and situational components are introduced. These result from events that occur without warning at a crucial time in an individual's development. Because of the untimely occurrence of the crisis, the individual may be delayed in achieving, or unable to achieve, certain developmental milestones.

The example selected here to illustrate a loss of mobility with both situational and developmental components is that of the adolescent male with a spinal cord injury. This hazardous event is listed on the grid under Loss of Sensory-Motor Exchange (see figure 6-3). The Loss of Mobility unit includes psychological immobility and chronicity. The writer chose the spinal cord injured client as an example because he illustrates these concepts as well as loss of physical mobility due to disruption of sensory motor functions. Several loss categories are usually involved in complex situations such as this, and integration is fostered by examples that demonstrate the interrelatedness of the various units of content.

The adolescent with a spinal cord injury is an appropriate example for the third level course because the crisis is precipitated by a sudden and unexpected event, the long-term outcome is unpredictable, accomplishment of developmental tasks is impeded, and the nursing interventions require a high level of knowledge and skill. Moreover, in dealing with this hazardous event, students must apply the knowledge of the nervous system, developmental theory, and loss of mobility gained in previous courses. They also use their knowledge of other loss categories, such as relationships and protective mechanisms. In addition they learn how to cope, and how to assist the client to cope with several new problems, depending on the level of the cord injury; for example, the possibility of permanent bilateral paralysis, bowel and bladder dysfunction, sexual dysfunction, a greater risk of skin breakdown, and the greater potential for respiratory complications.

Developmental considerations for the adolescent individual are particularly important because there are numerous tasks to be completed: establishing identity, achieving independence, forming intimate relationships, and selecting a career. Because of the serious nature of this event, the adolescent faces many changes in his life and has numerous obstacles to overcome in order to satisfactorily proceed with these developmental accomplishments. In order to cope successfully he must recognize and accept the decreased level of mobility and concomitant changes in body image. In addition, he needs acceptance of these changes from significant others. This previously mobile adolescent must accept some degree of dependence and the fact that he will view the remainder of his life from a wheelchair. Career goals, hobbies, and other meaningful activities may need altering. The impact on his sexual relationships may be profound.

As a basis for nursing interventions, both psychological and physical assessments are essential. These include identification of the individual's developmental level, his perception of the crisis, and his reaction to the long-term implications of his loss of mobility. Physical assessment of all body systems is needed but assessment of the skin, respiratory, and neuromuscular systems are of particular importance because of the nature of the injury.

The data gathered through these assessments are utilized in formulating a plan of care that will foster maximum growth. Such a plan includes helping the individual and family cope psychologically with the crisis. As important as the psychological care is the physical care that promotes healing and prevents complications.

Although students have learned many psychomotor skills during previous semesters, two new skills introduced at this level—tracheostomy care and suctioning—are particularly appropriate in this situation. If the spinal injury causes respiratory distress, these skills will be needed.

Communication skills are of special importance in collecting data and intervening successfully in this complex situation. Students have acquired basic communication skills in previous semesters but more sophisticated ones are introduced at this level; for example, developing a therapeutic relationship with a client in crisis. In addition, content of the process course focuses on the final step in the nursing process—evaluation.

The goal of nursing in this situation is to provide interventions that will lead to a positive resolution of the crisis. Students learn to identify the parameters of a positive resolution and to evaluate the individual's progress. In the biophysical realm, an intervention can be judged successful even if the body must sometimes function at a lower level of wellness than before the crisis. However, it should be possible to show growth in some area of the individual's functioning. These ideas are reflected in the following criteria for evaluating the effectiveness of the interventions for the adolescent with spinal cord injury: attaining and maintaining his maximum level of wellness; psychologically accepting his limitations; following his prescribed regime regarding diet, medications, follow-up care, physical care (such as skin care, bowel, and bladder regime), establishing positive relationships with peers, and successfully coping with new crises.

As patient outcomes are evaluated, needed changes in the plan of care are made. The individual as well as his family are included in this process as much as possible. Because of the chronicity factor inherent in this crisis, long-term goals become a significant part of the plan. Such planning must include preparation for rehabilitation, discharge to a rehabilitation setting or home, and teaching to promote health and prevent any complications related to immobility. An assessment of the home is a necessary part of the plan.

Students work with individuals coping with this type of crisis in a variety of settings. These include an acute care setting, a rehabilitation setting, and/or the individual's home. In any setting, past knowledge regarding the concepts of mobility, relationships, protective mechanisms, developmental needs, and the entire nursing process are applied. Psychomotor skills and intellectual skills learned throughout all nursing courses are incorporated appropriately to foster a positive resolution. It should be noted that students will work with clients that are similar from a nursing perspective to the one described here. The medical diagnoses, however, will vary widely.

To summarize, the concept of mobility in health and in illness has been traced through three levels of nursing courses. Initially, the focus is on the healthy individual. Next, the concept is expanded to include the implications of loss of mobility with the focus on illness. Finally, the concept is studied in a complex situation that includes developmental as well as biophysical/psychosocial considerations and encompasses several additional losses, integrating and correlating the crisis model and content.

THE SYNTHESIS SEMESTER

Study of the three stages of the crisis model and all steps of the nursing process is completed by the end of the seventh semester. The last semester process course provides the opportunity to synthesize the learning of the previous semesters through clinical application in an area of the student's choice; for example, biophysical or psychosocial crisis in an acute care setting or pre- and post-crisis in a community health setting. Students may also focus on a particular age group, for example, the child, or a particular type of hazardous event, for example, parenting. In this course, the time allotted to clinical laboratory is markedly increased. Class time is decreased and, in accordance with the grid, devoted to issues related to professional practice: interdependency, bureaucracy, accountability, management/leadership, consumer advocacy, and change agent.

The faculty's experience in developing the eighth semester process course, as compared to the three previous semesters, testifies to the usefulness of a conceptual model. For the first three semesters, the crisis theory formulation provided clear direction for course descriptions, objectives, and content. The courses offered in those three semesters have remained basically unchanged for seven years except for minor improvements and updating.

In contrast, the eighth semester process course entitled "A Synthesis of Theory and Practice in Nursing" has been debated and revised each year. Faculty have a clear understanding of the meaning of synthesis in nursing practice, so the clinical part of the course presents no problem. Faculty are less sure about the theory portion of the course, possibly because the relationship to the conceptual framework is not obvious.

The theory course is a seminar course in which students explore philosophical issues relevant to their practice. This course has worked well. In addition to helping students to formulate and articulate their beliefs about issues in health care, it provides an opportunity to practice the skills of group leadership and membership and to evaluate their peers.

SUMMARY

This chapter has described sample objectives and content for the four upper division semesters of a nursing curriculum. Much of the material presented here is undoubtedly familiar to the reader because it is similar to content included in a traditional curriculum. There is, after all, a body of facts and technical skills needed by all nurses in order to meet client needs.

What then is the difference? What makes the approach to nursing knowledge described in this book superior to the traditional design that focuses on medical specialties? One very obvious answer is that a design of this nature minimizes the duplication of content and compartmentalization of knowledge that characterized the old curriculum. However, the most meaningful response to the question is two-fold and transcends these issues. As pointed out previously, the crisis theory framework has provided faculty with effective direction for selecting and organizing content and learning experiences. More importantly, the framework provides the student—the professional practitioner of tomorrow—with direction and organization appropriate for all client situations at the care giving level. The following detailed explanation was excerpted from an unpublished paper by Eileen Murphy (1980) and is reproduced with the author's permission.

Use of the crisis theory framework identifies the parameters to be assessed in order to develop a data base for the planning of nursing care. Data need to be collected in order to identify the hazardous event, real or potential, and the precipitating factors leading to the event. The perception of the event held by the client and the meaning it has for him need to be examined, his habitual problem-solving behaviors identified, and their effectiveness in this situation assessed. Ineffective coping mechanisms that the client may be using need to be recognized, and internal and external resources, both needed and available, need to be considered.

As well as directing which data should be collected, the framework provides an excellent model for organizing the data. The crisis experience can be conceptualized in three stages: (a) pre-crisis stage, which would encompass all data relevant to precipitating factors, the hazardous event, the client's perceptions, his problem-solving attempts, and the results of these attempts; (b) the crisis stage, which would include data relevant to the cognitive and affective responses to the situation as well as the efforts taken to mobilize traditional resources; (c) the post-crisis stage, which would organize data relevant to crisis resolution, either positive or negative, in terms of levels of functioning

This organizational pattern suggests that the goals of nursing intervention can be described for each stage through the use of the levels of prevention concept (Shamansky and Clausen, 1980) which was contributed to crisis theory by the early public health collaborators. In the pre-crisis stage, the goal of nursing intervention would be to prevent the incidence of crisis, or primary prevention. During the crisis phase, the concept of secondary prevention defines the nursing goal as limiting the severity of the crisis. Finally, in the post-crisis phase, tertiary prevention emphasizes the goal of rehabilitation, or reaching the optimum level of functioning still possible.

Crisis theory cannot prescribe specific nursing interventions to meet these goals. However, as a framework, broad categorie of appropriate interventions can be identified. In the pre-crisis phase, nursing interventions would include efforts to reduce precipating factors that increase vulnerability to hazards, anticipatory guidance to enhance problem-solving skills, and reduction o the hazards inherent in some events.

Aguilera and Messick (1970) suggest three areas of nursing actions that seem most appropriate for the crisis phase: (a) interventions that help the client to perceive the problem realistically; (b) interventions to help the client to utilize appropriate and effective coping mechanisms; (c) interventions that serve to mobilize social supports and other external resources. Because of the emphasis on problem-solving, Barrell (1974) sees this framework identifying teaching activities in both the cognitive and affective domains as important nursing interventions.

In the post-crisis phase, nursing efforts are directed toward reinforcing the newly-learned problem-solving behaviors and exploring possible future application. In instances of unhealthy resolution, efforts can be directed toward maximizing the individual's functional potential and preventing major disorganization.

Evaluation activities specified by this framework address the extent to which new problem-solving behaviors have been learned and subsequently used in future appropriate situations. Other evaluative measures would be directed by the goals identified for the specific level of prevention being addressed.

The last chapter in this book, which was adapted from a paper written by a seventh semester student, illustrates the effectiveness of this approach to nursing. It is obvious that this student has internalized the crisis theory framework. She has learned a thought process that will guide her nursing actions in her future professional practice. Is that not the goal of professional nursing education?

7

The Laboratory Component

Dorothy Coburn
Evelyn Hayes
Pauline Hebert
Edna Johnson

Nursing education programs have traditionally included opportunities
for students to learn and to practice the skills of the profession in
addition to acquiring a body of cognitive knowledge. Early curricula
designated these activities "clinical experience" and included such
experience as an adjunct to nursing theory courses. As curriculum
designs became more sophisticated and the emphasis for clinical
activities focused on learning rather than on providing a service, the
terminology shifted from "experience" to "laboratory." The change
in terminology embodied substantive changes so that nursing laboratory now includes many of the components that characterize laboratories in other disciplines (Infante, 1975a). If used correctly,
laboratory is allotted credit according to a sound rationale, each
session has predetermined objectives appropriate to the course objectives, and laboratory activities are an integral part of a course
rather than an adjunct to it. [Infante has identified essential elements
of the laboratory concept (1975a).]

According to the philosophy of laboratory[*] developed by University of Connecticut faculty, laboratory activities are "designed to

---

[*]The University of Connecticut philosophy of laboratory was based on
the ideas developed by Mary Sue Infante in her doctoral dissertation
and later published (Infante, 1975a). The document, as it exists now,
reflects the input of numerous University of Connecticut faculty members and was accepted by faculty in 1977.

provide for transfer of knowledge from the theoretical situation to a simulated or real situation," (University of Connecticut School of Nursing, 1977, p. 64). Nursing laboratory includes two components: a laboratory in the college setting where students may learn and practice intellectual and psychomotor skills at their own pace; and clinical laboratory in which students apply learning from the college to a real life situation. This chapter describes the utilization of each of these components at the University of Connecticut, presents theory relative to psychomotor skill learning, and discusses the evaluation of clinical achievement.

THE COLLEGE LABORATORY

The college laboratory is comprised of two separate but closely related sections: the media laboratory and the simulation laboratory. The media laboratory houses self-instructional programs which can be listened to and viewed on an independent, student-paced basis. This activity can either enhance, complement, or replace reading materials or class content. The simulated laboratory houses equipment, models, mock-ups, and simulators which can be used and manipulated by students in learning the psychomotor and intellectual skills of nursing prior to actual patient contact in the clinical setting.

Simulated laboratory activities are integral components of the process courses and are reflective of the theoretical and process learnings undertaken during a particular semester. In the fall semester of the junior year, when students focus on assessment of individuals experiencing developmental hazardous events, simulated laboratory activities consist of physical assessment skills. In the spring semester of the junior year, when students progress to the planning and intervention phase of the nursing process, focusing on situational hazardous events, simulated laboratory activities consist of psychomotor skills used in nursing intervention appropriate for specific loss categories. In the senior year, when students are studying life-threatening crises, more complex psychomotor skills are included in the simulation laboratory learnings, for example, tracheostomy care, and care of chest tubes. The skills for all courses are listed on the grid.

Most of the psychomotor skills are learned during the fifth, sixth, and seventh semesters. As the student progresses to the eighth semester, the clinical laboratory time increases significantly since the student is now integrating all of the theories and skills previously learned. The time students spend in the simulation laboratory is therefore inversely related to clinical laboratory time; junior students spend more time in the simulation laboratory and senior students spend less time there.

Philosophy of College Laboratory

According to the philosophy of laboratory, the college laboratory provides students with an environment in which they may become active, self-paced learners. In this setting, students can experiment, investigate, and practice as their individual needs dictate, with a freedom to make errors apart from the clinical laboratory setting with its inherent demands and responsibilities. This safe and controlled simulated setting provides students with opportunities to learn to apply nursing theory to practice.

The college laboratory allows for greater freedom in individualizing a student's learning. This environment is also a means for achievement of course objectives which may not be otherwise achievable. In addition, it can also provide a setting for more precise means to evaluate skill learning.

Theories of Education for Psychomotor Skill Learning

Sensible educational practice mandates an appropriate meshing of educational strategy with learning objectives (Pittenger and Gooding, 1971). The University of Connecticut included statements about education and the teaching-learning process as components of the conceptual framework. In these statements, faculty expressed the belief that no single theory of learning is appropriate or applicable to all situations or for all types of objectives. The following brief comparison of associative learning theory with field theory supports this view. It is presented here because of its relevance to psychomotor skill learning—an area that the writer believes has been neglected in nursing education.

Morris Bigge (1976) describes an associative learning theory as any psychological theory that assumes learning is a process of combining or connecting ideas or actions in memory or behavior. He identifies stimulus-response conditioning theories as associative learning theories which belong in the behavioristic family of contemporary learning theories. Some of the more prominent stimulus-response (SR) conditioning theorists are Robert Gagne, Robert Glasser, and B. F. Skinner. Stimulus-response learning can promote memorization of a motor act's sequence (chaining the parts together to make a whole), so an associative learning model is useful in the college laboratory for psychomotor skill learning. However, this associative learning model will not further the philosophic aims of creative problem solving, investigation, and experimentation in the college laboratory.

A field theory of learning can be described as a cognitive learning theory which has grown out of Gestalt psychology (Bigge, 1976). Many of the psychological concepts in Gestalt psychology can be traced to Kurt Lewin's field psychology. Hilgard and Bower (1966) interpret the meaning of learning as used by Gestaltists, and later by cognitive-field theorists, as consisting of a reorganization or restructuring process within the learner's perceptual world, his field. Field theory is synonymous with configurational psychology and phenomenological or cognitive-field psychology. While cognitive-field theorists may differ on some points, they nevertheless share some common beliefs with one another and are more at odds with theorists in the behavioristic family of learning psychology. Some of the more active contributors to cognitive-field theory include Gordon Alport, Jerome Bruner, and John Dewey.

A theory of education utilized by a faculty should be compatible with the stated philosophy. The college laboratory philosophy emphasizes self-pacing, independent learning, experimentation, and investigation in problem solving. Therefore, field theory is appropriate to meet the objectives that flow from this philosophy. However, a field theory approach to motor skill learning seems to require an inordinate amount of time if the student is left alone and forced to figure out a particular motor skill chain for herself. Discovery learning is not the preferred method in this instance since it will result in student frustration and wasted time, with a concomitant delay in optimum learning. Therefore, in developing teaching strategies for the college laboratory, both the associative learning model and a field theory model should be utilized. The following discussion of a taxonomy for psychomotor skill learning adds another dimension for faculty consideration.

Taxonomies of Educational Objectives

The purposes of education have long been viewed by educators as encompassing three different domains of learning—cognitive, affective, and psychomotor. It has been stated previously that no single learning theory is appropriate for attainment of each and every learning objective. It is recognized also that no single learning theory is appropriate for all three domains since the outcomes and objectives for the separate domains will, of necessity, be different.

While a complete and arbitrary separation of the three domains is possible in theory, it usually fails in practice since educational objectives in one domain often overlap into the other two. For instance, a cognitive objective pertaining to knowledge of human anatomy could easily result in a student's deeper appreciation for the human body's ability to withstand physical stress; this affective domain objective may or may not have been identified in the course objectives, but its occurrence would be possible without purposeful consideration. This cross-effect is not limited to any one of the three domains. While attempting to provide educational experiences which will specifically fulfill an objective in one domain, a secondary objective, either identified or unidentified, may be achieved simultaneously, without intent, in another domain or even in the same one.

Curriculum and evaluation decisions have become more precise and the selection of learning experiences to satisfy end objectives has been greatly facilitated by the use of taxonomies. A taxonomy for the psychomotor domain is useful as an educational tool for consideration of knowledge acquired in the college laboratory since this is the setting of major importance for initial learning of psychomotor skills. Harrow (1972) describes categories for this domain similar to those developed for the cognitive domain (Bloom, 1956) and for the affective domain (Krathwohl, Bloom, and Masia, 1964).

The classification for psychomotor skill learning follows a pattern similar to the levels in Bloom's taxonomy for the cognitive domain. Bloom (1956) identifies knowledge and comprehension as being simpler behaviors than the more complex synthesis and evaluation behaviors. The more simple behaviors are, in fact, incorporated in the more complex behaviors.

> One may take the Gestalt point of view that the complex behavior is more than the sum of the simpler behaviors, or one may view the complex behavior as being completely analyzable into simpler components. But either way, so long as the simpler behaviors may be viewed as components of the more complex behaviors, we can view the educational process as one of building on the simpler behavior (Bloom, 1956, p. 16).

In the psychomotor taxonomy the same process occurs; for example, visual discrimination incorporates visual acuity, visual tracking, visual memory, figure ground differentiation, and perceptual consistency. Each classification level can be broken down to more specific detail for further analysis. Since the perceptual ability category is the most useful for nursing educators concerned with psychomotor skill learning, Harrow's breakdown of this category is presented below (Harrow, 1972, p. 87).

3.00 Perceptual Abilities
   3.10 Kinesthetic Discrimination
      3.11 Body Awareness
         3.111 Bilaterality
         3.112 Laterality
         3.113 Sidedness
         3.114 Balance
   3.20 Visual Discrimination
      3.21 Visual Acuity
      3.22 Visual Tracking
      3.23 Visual Memory
      3.24 Figure-Ground Differentiation
      3.25 Perceptual Consistency
   3.30 Auditory Discrimination
      3.31 Auditory Acuity
      3.32 Auditory Tracking
      3.33 Auditory Memory
   3.40 Tactile Discrimination
   3.50 Coordinated Abilities
      3.51 Eye-Hand Coordination
      3.52 Eye-Foot Coordination

Using Harrow's taxonomy, one can analyze any nursing skill for purposes of assessing its simplicity or complexity. For instance, passive range of motion exercises on a healthy postoperative patient can be classified as a simple psychomotor skill. If the individual is, instead, an acute severe arthritic with significant joint pathology the skill becomes more complex: finely attuned perceptual discriminations are called into play as the student attempts to identify the presence or absence of limited ranges of motion, muscle spasms, or joint crepitation. Taken further, the motor skill of percussion, according to Harrow's taxonomy, falls in the category of a coordinated ability since it involves two of the perceptual and/or movement patterns itemized in her classification scheme. For example, analysis of percussion skills reveal that eye-hand coordination of pleximeter and plexor fingers is involved as well as auditory discrimination of the resulting percussed sounds. The perceptual ability of auditory discrimination has been noted to include auditory acuity, auditory tracking, and auditory memory.

In summary, it can be noted that taxonomies might be useful to help faculty decide when a particular skill should be taught in a nursing curriculum based on the skill's simplicity or complexity. A taxonomy can also be used as a guide for realistic appraisal and expectation of student competencies; that is, whether a student can attain proficiency in learning a particular skill within a semester's time, for example, or whether it would be more realistic to expect proficiency in only one component of a complex skill within this time frame. Bloom states that a taxonomy's usefulness should lie in its ability to "provide a basis for suggestions as to methods for developing curricula, instructional techniques, and testing techniques" (1956, p. 21). The taxonomy of the psychomotor domain, as categorized by Harrow, clearly delineates the types of learning involved and provides a framework for analysis of tasks. Its use can facilitate the selection of instructional strategies for optimum learning and the subsequent selection of evaluative procedures to test learning. These ideas have not been utilized to any great extent at the University of Connecticut but they provide a challenging area for future development and research. Some examples of application to teaching are provided below.

Teaching Strategies for Psychomotor Skill Learnings

A clinical instructor recently entered a patient's room and found a junior nursing student preoccupied with changing a surgical abdominal dressing; the student was completely oblivious to the fact that the patient's intravenous tubing had become disconnected and was causing blood to spill onto the gown and bedclothes. The instructor later reprimanded the student for her negligence—was she blind? she asked. Needless to say, there was nothing wrong with the student's vision. What had occurred could be described as selective tunnel vision. The student was concentrating on seeing and attending to only the task at hand—the dressing change—while ignoring other important visual stimuli and information concerning the patient's clinical situation.

In any learning sequence there exists an apprehending phase, an acquisition phase, a storage phase, and a retrieval phase (Gagne, 1970). The apprehending phase is best described as a component of selective perception of stimuli with subsequent mental coding. The acquisition phase can be likened to the understanding process. The storage phase is either the long- or short-term memory aspect and the retrieval is the recall or transfer of the learning phase (Gagne, 1970).

The apprehending phase is of particular importance since it precedes the other phases in the learning sequence. If the student does not perceive the appropriate stimuli, learning cannot take place. This is of particular concern in sensory perceptual aspects of learning experiences. Haber (1969) researched visual perception abilities in an experiment with children; he found that they possessed an ability to see in great detail and that they could recall later, in equally great detail, elements of a picture previously viewed. He labelled this mental visual recall "eidetic imagery." While eight percent of the children in his sample possessed this ability, no adults did. Doob (1964) thinks that this deterioration in eidetic imagery (from childhood to adulthood) occurs because of society's demand that we store information verbally rather than visually.

What can be done to prevent students in the clinical setting from functioning with selective tunnel vision as shown in the previous example? One obvious suggestion is to improve the learning situation in the simulated laboratory so the student is prepared better for the clinical setting.

Psychomotor skill learning calls for different teaching strategies than those commonly used for teaching intellectual skills. Verbal transmission of information is no longer sufficient, for example. If the objective is to have the student learn a particular psychomotor skill sequence, the student must have an opportunity to see the skill being performed. Modeling is then possible as the student attempts to reproduce the actions visualized.

During this learning sequence, mental imagery comes into play since the student tries to match motor skill performance to the recalled memory pattern. If the objective is to have the student discriminate between breath sounds, the teaching methodology must be geared to provide the student with auditory experiences that can be listened to and learned for later identification and recognition. Simulated perceptual sensory experiences must be incorporated in the learning experience to provide the learner with a frame of reference for later recognition and identification.

Another aid to learning in the simulated laboratory setting is feedback of results during practice. This serves to reinforce correct action, motivating and rewarding the student; this reinforcement increases the probability that the specific behavior will be repeated in the future. The learning atmosphere should be relaxed and supportive since high anxiety levels have been proven to be detrimental to psychomotor skill performance (Weiner, 1959).

The instructional exchange between the instructor and the student generates additional stress for the student which can influence psychomotor performance. Verbal comments should be made either before or after but not during the actual motor performance. A student learning a new motor skill must attend to the task at hand and cannot process simultaneous auditory stimuli. These stimuli tend to be blocked by the student, requiring later repetition (Greer, Hitt, Sitterley, and Slobodnick, 1972).

The above suggestions can result in a greater increase in learning in the simulated laboratory setting. Either mediated or simulated exercises can be created specifically to sharpen visual perceptive abilities. Additionally, if Haber's findings related to eidetic imagery are truly representative of adult abilities, then the implications for nursing curricula are significant, implying that educators need to focus on ways to redevelop this lost ability. If creative ways are developed for increasing learning in the college laboratory, the student will have less need to concentrate so completely when performing a psychomotor skill in the clinical setting and can, therefore, attend to additional stimuli which are peripheral to the task at hand.

Some additional points should be made about the selection and use of instructional media. This teaching aid has been demonstrated to be effective in numerous research studies. Without it, student self-pacing would not be possible. The most important criterion for the selection and utilization of media is the program's ability to satisfy one or more of the course objectives. Yet, a survey of colleges in the state of New York showed that "rarely . . . was there a widely shared, coherent rationale for the use of instructional technology. In only a few colleges was it regarded as part of a system of teaching . . . rooted in clearly articulated objectives and principles of learning" (Richards, 1974, p. 482).

The appropriate and timely use of instructional technology requires more faculty preparation time than traditional forms of instruction. The media program must be previewed by faculty to determine if it is relevant to course objectives. If it is found to be appropriate, a decision must be made as to whether the program will be integrated into a lecture or seminar, used to supplement class content as needed or desired by students, or used independently for student self-instruction. Additional consideration must also be given to methods of incorporating the content covered by media formats into the examination materials by which students are evaluated.

Used alone or in combination with class presentations and/or clinical experiences media programs can: facilitate the comprehension of theory; assist students in the application of theory to nursing practice; provide students with modeling for learning step-by-step sequences of nursing psychomotor skills; assist in refreshing or reviewing such previously learned supportive scientific knowledge as anatomy and physiology; provide students with simulated clinical observations which may not be encountered in the real clinical situation; and provide students with simulated practice exercises to enhance such sensory observational skills as visual, tactile, and auditory observations for patient assessment.

The anticipated values of the college laboratory as stated in the philosophy have been partly realized at the University of Connecticut. The use of media has allowed for student self-pacing, freed class time for higher-level learning, and enabled laboratory staff to devote more time to individualized instruction and feedback in the simulated laboratory. Students view media then practice skills at their own pace and as often as needed to achieve the required competence. Staff are available as a resource. In providing guidance when the student requests it, the staff member helps the student to identify and correct her own errors and explore variations in techniques for hypothetical situations.

To date, very little attention seems to have been given to encourage the student to be creative. Neither has the potential of laboratory activities to develop clinical judgment been realized. Much greater use could be made of media for remedial instruction, for problem-solving activities, and for innovative, creative approaches to learning nursing tasks. In order for this to happen, faculty need time to think creatively, to identify programs which can meet the described needs, to develop new programs, and to conduct research on the effectiveness of various teaching strategies. This should include research on the application of educational theory and Harrow's taxonomy of objectives to psychomotor skill learning.

As with any instructional strategy, the length of time it has been in use has a relationship to progress in the field. Viewed on a developmental continuum, nursing faculty's expertise with instructional media can be said to be in the infancy stage. While instructional technology is not novel, much work remains to be done before its use can become maximized. Many of the faculty at the University of Connecticut recognize this undeveloped potential. A faculty task force for the development of instructional modules has been in existence for several years and results are hoped for in the not too distant future.

Operationalizing the Philosophy of College Laboratory

According to the philosophy of laboratory, when students go to the clinical setting they are fully prepared for the activities they will perform. Part of this preparation is the acquisition of the needed psychomotor skills. Faculty have identified essential skills and developed study guides for them. The study guide includes the objectives of the skill, selected readings, media programs, appropriate problem-solving activities, and a list of critical elements that are used for assessing competence. These materials are distributed at the beginning of the semester.

In keeping with the philosophy of self-pacing, students are responsible for organizing their work and completing the required activities within specified time limits. Initially, this time limit was the end of the semester. Faculty subsequently found it necessary to establish deadlines dispersed throughout the semester. In a given week, a student may choose to complete several skills or none, depending upon individual needs.

After considerable trial and error, a random type of sign-up system was established for student practice sessions. (Students draw numbers to determine the order for selection of practice time.) This system provides each student with a guaranteed practice time each week. Students may opt not to practice at this time, thereby releasing it for a classmate or they may request additional time if it is needed. Students are expected to either keep appointments or notify laboratory staff when they cannot, an expectation which promotes the development of accountability. This system has proven to be much more feasible than the system of complete freedom that was established initially.

As a preparation for practice, students are expected to follow the steps in the study guide. Laboratory personnel are available as a resource during each practice session but students are not permitted to use the staff as a substitute for independent study. When a student feels ready, he or she makes an appointment for evaluation.

The tool for evaluating skill performance is the list of critical elements included in the student's study guide. The elements are organized in a logical, step-wise fashion, proceeding from the first to the last component of the skill. These critical elements are written in very precise terms that clearly identify exactly what is expected of the student. If he or she misses a critical element, the evaluation session is terminated. After additional study and practice, another appointment is scheduled.

Activities evaluated in the college laboratory are graded on a pass/fail basis. All students are expected to complete assigned activities before the end of the semester. Failure to complete them results in a grade of F or Incomplete in the process course. Incomplete grades are subject to the usual university regulations.

Some of the problems experienced in operating the laboratory center around student scheduling and insufficient space, equipment, and media. Because of these factors many students have college laboratory activities in the evening, at the end of a busy day which has included clinical laboratory in the morning and classes in the afternoon. A schedule of this nature is stressful and can hamper a student's ability to concentrate, affecting his ability to learn. It has been demonstrated in research studies that psychomotor skill performance drops markedly with fatigue (Greer, Hitt, Sitterley, and Slobodnick, 1972). In light of this factor, the faculty should analyze student schedules and work load to see if expectations are realistic. Some students have elected to lighten the class load by taking some of the non-nursing courses during the summer.

In addition to the scheduling problem, the limited number of models, mock-ups, and simulators, due to financially stringent conditions, has limited the effectiveness of the simulated laboratory. Moreover, there is an absence of simulators available on the commercial market to adequately teach certain nursing skills. The large numbers of students using the in-house equipment causes rapid wearing and breakage of simulators and models, resulting in additional costs for repair or replacement. These factors are probably unavoidable and should be considered in the planning for a college laboratory.

Another problem has been staffing. One aspect of this is the difficulty in finding baccalaureate-prepared nurses who are skilled in physical assessment and who are interested in a position in a college laboratory. Lacking qualified applicants, the solution has been extensive in-service training. Even then, the position tends to be used as a stepping stone to other career goals, resulting in a high staff attrition rate. This problem has been circumvented to some degree by hiring graduate assistants—students currently in the graduate nursing program who have already learned physical assessment. While these graduate assistants have the necessary skills, they bring different perspectives with them regarding the role of physical assessment skills in nursing. Prepared at the graduate level with skills for screening and management, but not prepared for teaching, they have difficulty in adjusting their perspective to the undergraduate level where assessment skills are used as a basis for nursing interventions and not for primary care.

Another aspect of the staffing problem stems from a philosophical issue that is still unresolved. This will be discussed in Chapter 8. In spite of these problems, the college laboratory has been basically successful and it is a permanent part of the program. This phase of learning is a crucial step in preparing for clinical laboratory activities.

THE CLINICAL LABORATORY

Philosophy of Clinical Laboratory

According to the philosophy, the clinical laboratory provides client contact for the student for the purpose of integrating previously acquired knowledge and skills and applying them to real situations. Client contact is utilized when objectives cannot be met in the classroom or in the college laboratory. There is a progressive aspect to clinical study in that students first learn to apply knowledge to selected aspects of care and then later learn to give comprehensive care to clients. It is in the clinical laboratory (which may be an institution, a home, or the community) that the student develops clinical judgment in all phases of the nursing process and learns, through participation, how to be a contributing team member.

To operationalize the philosophy of clinical laboratory, guidelines were written for students, faculty, and agency personnel. These guidelines help to clarify protocol, responsibilities, and lines of communication. Both the philosophy and guidelines clearly indicate that clinical activities are to be planned with stated objectives and that faculty should guide rather than supervise students; students may therefore be in a clinical laboratory without the presence of a faculty advisor. This policy has proven controversial for some clinical agencies and for some of the faculty. The idea of students in the clinical setting without faculty was a complete departure from the norm. It has been acceptable for some clinics and non-medically oriented agencies such as schools, day-care centers, and senior citizen centers. Hospitals, however, have wanted faculty present for students' activities; some even insisted that student experience in such specialized settings as pediatrics and maternity be under the guidance of faculty with masters' degrees and experience in those areas. It has therefore been necessary to carefully negotiate contracts so that the needs and integrity of both the agency and the school can be met and maintained.

Early in the development of the philosophy of laboratory it was envisioned that, in any given week, students would go to a variety of settings, at variable hours, in pursuit of individualized learning activities. Agencies have placed some constraints on this; economic factors have placed yet another constraint. With the escalation of gasoline prices, it has become unrealistic to expect students to drive twenty to thirty miles in order to perform isolated activities of short duration. One might perhaps challenge the validity of allowing such a nonacademic factor to influence the structure of learning activities, but it is well-known that consideration of the learner's needs and reduction of stress factors have a positive influence on learning.

Since faculty came from traditional programs, both in terms of their professional studies and their teaching experiences, adaptation of clinical expectations to an integrated program was problematic. There was a tendency to try to include all the elements of the more traditional programs into the new one. Furthermore, professional expectations of the state licensing body and the profession itself added other pressures, particularly on the student.

In reaction to these pressures, the faculty identified and described the essential laboratory learnings. This helped not only to operationalize the philosophy and the crisis theory framework, but also to create more realistic expectations of student activities. At the level meetings, faculty in the various regions shared how specific learnings were being realized. It was and continues to be necessary to have interlevel meetings to monitor the integrity and flow of clinical activities.

The Junior Level

Some of the required junior level clinical learning experiences are allocated to a specific semester. Others may take place any time during the year. Emphasis is on the meeting of level objectives, not on setting or time. However, the allocation of three credits for laboratory assumes a minimum of nine clinical hours per week.

In the fifth semester courses, the focus is on pre-crisis, the concept of wellness throughout the life span, and the skills needed to assess the health of clients at each developmental level, including the complete childbearing cycle. Therefore, clinical laboratory activities are designed to provide opportunities for students to use assessment techniques in interactions with well clients. They collect data by observation, interviewing, and physical assessment, then analyze the data and draw conclusions. Client problems and strengths are analyzed and, ultimately, a nursing diagnosis formulated.

At the junior level, the required experiences have been incorporated into a student record form that includes the theoretical base for each experience and examples of activities, the settings that can be used to meet the requirement, and whether it can take place in either semester. Students note the date of each experience along with appropriate comments (see figure 7-1).

Each faculty member explores her geographic region to identify the clinical resources that can provide the types of experience that have been identified as essential. This involves matching the time the experiences are available with the students' schedules and negotiating details of the experience with the agencies. This negotiation usually includes the students' role, the time commitment of the agency, and such details as the availability of parking and student dress.

The faculty member identifies specific objectives for each laboratory experience. These objectives and guidelines for the experience are given to students. In addition, the students formulate at least one objective for their own learning; this helps them to become actively involved.

An example of a clinical laboratory experience provided for some students in the fifth semester takes place at a senior citizens' nutrition center. The clients come to the center for the noon meal, arriving at least an hour before the meal to allow time for social interaction. In this setting, students perform a mental health assessment and the observation component of physical assessment, using the appropriate study guides as a basis for their activities. This provides an opportunity to assess an essentially well elderly person and have first hand experience with content included in the theory course, that is, changing physical status and adaptation to socialization as it relates to the elderly individual. After the experience, the students record and analyze their findings, compare them with norms, identify strengths and weaknesses, and arrive at a nursing diagnosis.

The faculty member is not present in the agency during this experience. However, the written care plan is reviewed by the faculty member and appropriate feedback is given to the student. This is done in writing and also verbally during individual and group clinical conferences.

In this semester students begin the Family Study described in Chapter 4. All students select a family and begin to establish a relationship with the family and with individual family members. A few students may begin to gather data for the assessments that are required to be completed before the end of the junior year.

Required Experiences	Theoretical Base	Activities	Representative Hazardous Events
Care of a client experiencing Loss of Regulation	N223 Loss of Fluid and Electrolytes Loss of Neurological Regulation Loss of Hormonal Regulation Loss of Respiratory Patency Loss of Cellular Regulation N228 Planning and Intervention Principles of Body Mechanics Principles of Medication & I.V. Administration Care of the Client Experiencing Surgery	Assessment, Planning, Intervention with Adult or Child Experiencing Real or Threatened Loss of Regulation Suggested Activities Cardiovascular Assessment Respiratory Assessment Neurological Assessment Other Appropriate Assessments Admin.-meds, I.V.'s, O_2 Monitoring Health Teaching Sugar, Acetone Testing Participation in I.V. Therapy Observation Diagnostic/ Therapeutic Radiology Procedures Observation Pulmonary Function Tests Observation/Participation in Oncology Program (Rounds, Conferences, etc.) Investigation/Utilization Specific Community Resources Surgical Follow-through Follow-up Care (Discharge Planning, Home Visits, Clinics)	Development of Edema State of Dehydration Occurrence of Hypovolemic Shock Alteration in Insulin Regulation Alteration in Thyroid Regulation Alteration in Adrenocortical Regulation Presence of Respiratory Infection Development of Atelectasis Occurrence of Benign Neoplasms Occurrence of Malignant Neoplasms Hyperactivity in Children

FIGURE 7-1. Excerpt from Junior Level Experience Record. The form includes columns for the student to enter the date of the experience plus comments.

It should be noted that all students do not have identical experiences. There are, for example, a variety of resources that provide opportunities for students to interact with elderly clients and perform the activities described in the illustration. At the end of each semester all clinical laboratory experiences are evaluated by faculty to determine their effectiveness in meeting the established objectives. This is done jointly with students and agency personnel. While the evaluation with the agency is informal and usually verbal, students are expected to submit a formal evaluation of each of their experiences. Changes for subsequent semesters are based on the outcomes of these evaluations.

In the sixth semester clinical laboratory experiences provide the opportunity for students to practice their skills of data collection, analysis, and formulation of a nursing diagnosis with clients experiencing a situational hazardous event. In addition, they learn the process of planning and intervention and a variety of psychomotor skills. Clinical laboratory experiences now include integrative activities rather than just the singular activities characteristic of the preceding semester.

Students continue the Family Study initiated in the previous semester by doing a complete developmental assessment on each family member and by anticipating the developmental hazardous events. Data are gathered for family and neighborhood assessments. By the end of the semester, the student is expected to have determined strengths, potential health problems, and a nursing diagnosis for each family member as well as for the family as a unit.

During this semester, each student is required to have an experience with a depressed client (loss of relationships) in any type of setting; with a hospitalized client experiencing loss of mobility; and with clients in any type of setting experiencing loss of regulation, loss of sensory motor exchange, and loss of protection. Another required experience is the surgical cycle which subsumes several loss categories—regulation, protective mechanisms, mobility, relationships, and, possibly, sensory-motor exchange. In order that a variety of developmental levels be included, all students must have experience with hospitalized children and with an elderly client in the home, hospital, or nursing home. The specific focus for each type of experience and the theoretical base are noted on the experience record.

The student completes the process of assessment, planning, and intervention for each client. Although evaluation is primarily a senior activity, junior students begin to learn this final step of the nursing process. In addition, they are expected to make at least two home visits after discharge of at least one of their hospitalized clients. Specific guidelines have been developed for each type of experience to supplement the activities listed on the experience record.

In selecting experiences, the faculty member considers not only the loss category but also the opportunity to practice essential psychomotor skills. (These are identified on the experience record.) The selection for an individual student depends upon that student's readiness. Because of the philosophy of self-pacing, the requirement that a student first demonstrate competence in the college laboratory, and the limitations of space and time in the laboratory, students are at varying levels of achievement at any given time. This factor influences faculty planning.

Another constraint that influences the selection of clinical laboratory experiences is the availability of the desired client situations. For example, some of the smaller community hospitals have a limited number of postoperative clients on any given day. On the other hand, in the large hospitals with active surgical services many students use the same units.

There are several ways of dealing with these disparate factors. One is by careful sequencing of content. For example, the unit on loss of mobility is scheduled quite early in the semester. Many clients in acute care hospitals and extended care facilities are experiencing this loss, so it is relatively easy to select appropriate learning situations for all students. Some of these clients require only a limited number of psychomotor skills and others need many. This factor facilitates selection of a client appropriate to each student's level of readiness. Planning experiences in the late afternoon or evening is another way to find the required activity and avoid the hours when an agency is congested with many students and personnel.

The surgical cycle, because of its integrative nature both in terms of theoretical content and psychomotor skills, is scheduled late in the semester. This gives most students time to have completed the college laboratory activities. Ideally, a client who is one day postoperative following abdominal surgery is selected for the experience. The student is expected to use assessment skills, especially physical assessment of the abdomen and the cardiorespiratory system as well as assessment of pain and fluid and electrolyte balance. A convenient time for this activity is late afternoon and early evening. With faculty guidance, the student gathers the appropriate data while providing evening care to the client. From this data a nursing diagnosis and plan of care are formulated. The student is thus prepared to implement the plan the following morning, to evaluate the results, and make suggestions for revisions.

For all clinical experiences, the faculty member guides the student by asking questions that help her to see relationships between concepts. The student is encouraged to problem-solve while providing care. The faculty member provides immediate feedback to the student on the performance of technical skills and, additionally, reviews all written care plans and provides written feedback on each plan.

The student and faculty advisor meet frequently to discuss progress and identify learning needs. The completed experience record is reviewed at the end of the semester to identify areas that need strengthening. The record is passed along to the senior year clinical advisor, who uses it to assist the student in establishing goals for the seventh semester.

The Senior Level

The philosophy of laboratory indicates that, as the student progresses through the program, clinical laboratory experiences increase as college laboratory decreases. Therefore, in the senior year, laboratory experiences are predominantly clinical. Since the objectives and structure of the clinical component are not the same for the two semesters, each semester will be discussed individually.

The student comes to the senior year having worked with clients experiencing a developmental or a situational hazardous event. In the first semester of the senior year the focus is on interventions with clients experiencing combined events which place them in or at high risk for crisis. The student spends approximately 12 hours a week in an acute care setting, the setting where clients in crisis are most readily available. Since classroom instruction provides the student with concepts related to evaluation and the more complex assessment and intervention skills necessary for crisis situations, the student is expected to apply the total nursing process to selected clients.

Client selection is made by the student with appropriate guidance from the faculty advisor and agency staff. The student has to consider all of the loss categories relevant to each client, although the plan of care may be concentrated on one loss. At least once during the semester, the student must work with a client from each age group and deal with each loss category as highest priority. Throughout this semester emphasis is placed on the last two stages of the crisis model—crisis and crisis resolution.

As the student learns in the theory course about selected crises relative to each loss category, attempts are made to select concurrent clinical activities to which these concepts can be applied. Given the time constraints of a semester, the large number of students, and the restricted availability of certain types of experience, this is not always possible. This does not present a problem for those students who study loss of patency in September and have clients who experience those losses, such as cardiopulmonary or gastrointestinal obstructions, in November. However, it does present a problem for those students working with clients experiencing losses which have not yet been addressed in the theory course, such as the client withdrawn from reality or the high-risk mother. In these situations the faculty advisor must provide more direct clinical guidance.

Prior to those hours designated for clinical laboratory, the student is expected to go to the agency and select a client appropriate to her learning needs. Data are collected from assessments of client, the client's record, and staff. The student then designs a plan of care and reviews theory and skills relevant to that plan. Following the implementation of the plan the student must submit a written account which includes subjective, objective, and developmental data, analysis, nursing diagnoses, plan, nursing interventions, evaluation of client response, and self-evaluation.

The acute care setting is not the only clinical laboratory utilized in this semester. To find the client at risk for loss of reproductive integrity, students may go to clinics for high-risk mothers. Some students find this client through personal sources. Involvement with these clients has ranged from a one time contact to regular contacts through labor and delivery. The focus is on risk factors rather than the normal process of this developmental event.

The community component at this time focuses primarily on crisis resolution. Students may contract with clients in this third stage of crisis either through home visits of clients seen in the hospital or structured experience with a community health agency. Students are expected to assist clients to utilize those resources available to them and to reinforce clients' strengths.

Finally, students continue to make monthly visits to their study families. They continue with health assessments and health teaching as indicated as well as with neighborhood assessment for analysis of the ability of a given community to meet the health needs of a specific family. The senior level objectives for the Family Study as well as assessment tools guide these activities.

There are some variations in the manner in which faculty guidance is provided. Some faculty have chosen to provide all of the guidance for their individual groups of students. This involves faculty movement in and out of selected settings and a generalist rather than specialist approach to clinical teaching. Other faculty have formed teams of two or three, each providing guidance in her particular area of expertise, while students move through different settings. Another system which has been employed by a few faculty is an "on-off" system. To accommodate large groups of students and limited agency resources, clinical groups are divided in half and the subgroups then utilize the agency on alternate weeks. Related activities, such as follow-up visits, are planned for the unscheduled weeks. Research is needed to compare and evaluate the merits of all of these approaches.

Students frequently experience this semester as, indeed, one of crisis, not only for their clients but also for themselves. Time, energy, and resources are taxed as the student meets the demands of a frequently changing clinical experience. Students are held accountable for acquiring all essential learnings and faculty need to support them in their quests and assist them to find viable options. Both faculty and students welcome the advent of the eighth semester.

This final semester is a synthesis semester, and the clinical course offers the student an opportunity to gain indepth experience in an area of her choice. The selection process occurs in the seventh semester when faculty present an outline of the learning activities and modalities provided in selected settings representing pre-crisis, crisis, and/or post-crisis. Students then identify their first, second, and third choices. The majority of students receive their first choice. The very few, approximately four to five percent, who only get their third choice have their specialty area but not their preferred setting.

With a minimum of 18 hours in the clinical laboratory, students are able to become involved in the total spectrum of client care. As they apply and refine the skills which have been developing over the past three semesters, they become more secure in their professional identities. Students are expected to demonstrate nursing practice that brings together theoretical and experiential learning, incorporating leadership, and reflecting the standards of the profession.

Furthermore, they are expected to analyze the care setting in relation to the concepts being taught in class which are change, advocacy, management, and legality.

Students have expressed highly positive feelings toward this semester. They feel competent and appreciated, and their self-confidence increases. In some settings it is easy for the student to become service oriented and it may be necessary to reinforce the student role. Faculty then assist the student in valuing and applying both crisis theory and the nursing process in the "real" situation.

EVALUATING CLINICAL ACHIEVEMENT

The evaluation of student achievement in the clinical setting, like all evaluation, presents a challenge, but one which is even greater because this evaluation provides the basis for determining an individual's competence to practice, and the certification of this competence is a grave responsibility. Issues in evaluation, the school's philosoph of evaluation, and the major components of the evaluation process are addressed below.

Issues in Evaluation

Several concerns are inherent in any discussion of evaluation. Primary questions to be answered by a faculty are: Should evaluation be criterion-based or normative-referenced? Should laboratory be letter graded or merely rated pass/fail? Each of these questions will be addressed.

Criterion-referenced versus Formative-referenced. The University of Connecticut faculty needed more information before they could answer the above question. The curriculum project evaluator therefore researched the subject and prepared the comparison presented in figure 7-2. The evaluation task force studied the analysis and presented it to the faculty with a recommendation that the following points be accepted: 1) emphasis on student achievement of behavioral objectives, 2) deemphasis on competition between students, 3) orientation toward criterion-referenced measurement.

During discussion it became apparent that the faculty felt strongly that there were identifiable behaviors expected of every student for each course. Furthermore, objectivity, validity, and reliability

Criterion	Normative
Learner's behavior is compared to behavioral objectives	One student is compared to other students Norms are based on group frequencies -rank order student -normal bell-shaped curve is desired (in instrument development)
Well-suited for process curriculum where individual instruction and active involvement of learner is stressed	Does not allow as much feedback and growth
Establish quantitative and qualitative levels of mastery	Aspect of finality promotes chance of failure
Decreases student competition and facilitates cooperative learning and mutual support groups	Fosters independent, isolated achievement
Students can assume responsibility for helping each other because the other's achievement does not influence his grade	Student is penalized for helping peers; he conceals knowledge, guards information. Competition is promoted
Meaningfulness of an individual score is not dependent on comparison with other testees	Meaningfulness of an individual's score emerges from comparison with scores of others
This is suitable when we are interested in whether an individual possesses a particular skill, and there are no limits on how many people may possess that skill. Best technique for monitoring a student's passage through a curriculum and for deciding if he/she can pass to a more advanced level. Also, this is the best method for making judgments about curriculum or teaching methods employed	Comparison with other individuals is appropriate in decisions concerning selection or placement (granting of special awards or privileges, graduate school admissions, job references)

FIGURE 7-2. Comparison of criterion-referenced and normative-referenced evaluation.

in measurement were identified as desirable qualities for all aspects of the evaluation process. The faculty therefore voted to use criterion-referenced rather than normative-referenced techniques for clinical evaluation.

To Grade or Not to Grade Clinical Achievement. The issue of grading clinical laboratory was more difficult to resolve. Faculty disagreed on whether clinical evaluation should be a weighted portion of the total course grade or be graded on a pass/fail basis. Factors considered that supported the weighted letter grade included:

1. Clinical achievement cannot be reflected on the student's transcript unless it is assigned a letter grade and it is not possible to combine a letter grade and a pass/fail grade. (Clinical laboratory does not constitute a course in itself, but is allocated a portion of the credits in each clinical course.)
2. Grades are motivating factors for students (Hales, Bain, & Rand, 1973).
3. Pass/fail implies expectation of minimum level of competence, and faculty favor support of other than minimal standards.
4. Various levels of acceptable (pass) behavior can be identified and acknowledged by assigning a grade.
5. The literature indicates that in a pass/fail system, students do not achieve to capacity (Harrington, 1974; Hales, Bain, & Rand, 1973; Stuckley & Cook, 1976). The pass/fail system is, therefore, in contradiction to the school's conceptual framework in which facilitating optimum growth is a prominent feature.

Factors considered that supported the pass/fail system included:

1. Open communication between students and faculty may be diminished when grades are assigned. Pass/fail "reduces the threat of evaluation for the students. It tends to reduce significantly the academic games usually played between faculty and students. Instead, both faculty and students are now working together toward common goals" (Litwack, Sakata, & Wykle, 1972, p. 144).
2. An element of subjectivity is inherent in clinical evaluation. It is easier to discriminate between two levels of performanc (pass/fail) than five levels of performance (A to F).

As the pros and cons of grading clinical achievement were being considered, some of the discussion centered on methods of weighting the clinical grade. Two options were suggested: 1) weighting of clinical grade to be based on the proportion of course hours (credits) devoted to clinical laboratory; and 2) weighting of clinical grade to be determined for each course by faculty teaching that cours

After issues related to evaluation of student achievement in the clinical laboratory had been identified, small group discussions were held so that faculty could share thoughts, rationale, and questions. As with other aspects of curriculum development, this process facilitated understanding of each issue as well as the interrelationships among issues. Finally, at a meeting of the total faculty, a consensus was reached on grading achievement in all clinical courses except the first one. At the present time, the nature of the clinical activities in the fifth semester has made it difficult to distinguish clear levels of performance. Therefore, students are graded pass/fail on the basis of completing all clinical assignments and passing the critical elements of each assessment performed in the college and clinical laboratories. The possibility of reconsidering this decision is being discussed however.

Philosophy of Evaluation

As faculty were debating evaluation issues it became apparent that decisions were reflective of faculty beliefs and that these beliefs should be incorporated into a statement of philosophy of evaluation. It was also recognized that such a philosophy should be congruent with the school's philosophy and the conceptual framework. Such a statement was therefore drafted by a task group and accepted by faculty.

Faculty beliefs about evaluation are consistent with the crisis theory conceptual framework. For example, growth is a prominent feature of the crisis theory model, and the following statements from the philosophy support that goal:

> The evaluation process insures that the learner is provided with unique and relevant experiences for growth. . . . The learner understands the evaluation process and participates in his/her own evaluation. . . . The evaluation process provides both the teacher and learner with evidence concerning strengths and weaknesses. The faculty believes that the evaluation process is essential for the learner's growth. . . . The learner participates in the evaluation process. . . . [University of Connecticut School of Nursing, 1975, p. 56.]

All of these statements indicate that faculty view evaluation as a learning process and agree with Rogers that "learning is facilitated

when the student participates responsibly in the learning process"
(1969, p. 162). Moreover, such participation is essential to foster
personal growth. Another example of congruence between the conceptual framework and the philosophy of evaluation is the emphasis
on identification of the student's strengths and weaknesses and the
provision of "unique and relevant experiences for growth."

The philosophy of evaluation expresses the faculty's belief that
evaluation of students is a systematic, ongoing process which determines at what level the learner achieves in relation to predetermined
objectives, and that the evaluation process is built on the following
six components: 1) developing specific objectives; 2) developing
evaluative tools to determine achievement of the objectives; 3) determining the validity and reliability of the evaluation tools; 4) gathering data; 5) critically interpreting data and assigning scores on the
basis of outcomes; and 6) constructively communicating the results
to those concerned. Each of these components will now be illustrated.

Developing Specific Objectives

The course objectives are congruent with the philosophy of evaluation, which states that: "Objectives are written in the form of expected outcomes that are observable behaviors." This first component of the evaluation process-developing specific objectives—is of
prime importance to the process. Predetermined objectives mandate
the provision of relevant knowledge and experiences. In addition,
they ensure that all learners are evaluated by the same criteria. To
illustrate, a representative segment of the clinical objectives, specifically those associated with the planning phase of the nursing process
is given below. These objectives relate to the crisis model and
demonstrate progression from one level to the next.

6th semester
    2.0 Designs a plan of intervention utilizing the component parts
        of planning for an individual/family experiencing a hazardous
        event or crisis.
        2.1 Identifies the problem(s) of the individual/family.
        2.2 Identifies the strength(s) of the individual/family.
        2.3 Sets priorities for identifying the problem(s) of the
            individual family.
        2.4 States the rationale for priority listing of problems.

2.5 Formulates mutual long- and short-term behavioral objectives for the identified problem(s).

2.6 Develops a written plan for the identified problem(s).

7th semester

2.0 Designs plans appropriate for client/family/community.

2.1 Writes objectives and outcome criteria in measurable terms.

2.2 Confirms plans with client and family.

2.3 Establishes priorities for interventions.

2.4 Communicates plan to appropriate others.

8th semester

1.0 Designs individualized nursing care plans for clients and/ or families which reflect a focus on all actual and potential health problems.

1.1 Collects a complete data base which reflects data from an assessment of the client, his family, and/or significant others, and from previous or concurrent assessments conducted by other health team members.

1.2 Analyzes the data to differentiate between normal and abnormal bio-psycho-social behaviors.

1.3 After formulating a comprehensive list, deals with the problems according to priority.

1.4 Writes behavioral objectives with specific outcome criteria for each problem in consultation with the client/family.

1.5 Identifies nursing interventions which have a high probability for success in achieving the established outcome criteria.

1.6 Communicates the plan of care to all care providers.

Developing Evaluative Tools

Developing evaluative tools to determine achievement of the objectives is the second aspect of the evaluation process. The tool for evaluating college laboratory activities by means of critical elements has been described earlier. Clinical evaluation is much broader in scope and requires a different type of tool. Since the objectives of courses with a clinical component follow a standard format that coincides with the steps in the nursing process, the evaluation tool has a similar design. It comprises four sections—assessment, planning, intervention, and evaluation.

The above representative sample of objectives can be seen to be too global to be used effectively for evaluation. In order to be useful for evaluation, an objective must be very specific and be broken down into components. Therefore, for each clinical objective, faculty developed a list of cue behaviors which facilitate the students' understanding and fulfillment of the objectives.

Cue behaviors operationalize the objectives; they describe some student behaviors to be demonstrated to meet an objective. They are examples of behaviors and are not all inclusive. Some are so crucial that all students are required to demonstrate them; others are optional or not applicable in all situations. Students are also encouraged to be creative in seeking ways to meet an objective. For example, the eighth semester subobjective 1.4, "Writes behavioral objectives with specific outcome criteria for each problem in consultation with the client/family," has as cue behaviors the following: writes long- and short-term behavioral objectives; plans realistic goals in terms of available resources; changes goals appropriately; and evaluates client's/family involvement in outcome criteria.

The philosophy of evaluation states: "The measurement of both quantitative and qualitative achievement of an objective is accomplished through the use of established levels of performance (critical elements) for each objective. The levels of performance establish the degrees of competency necessary for achievement of an objective." In other words, behaviors have been identified which discriminate levels of performance and are reflected in the grading system. In addition, each level has been assigned a value from 0 to 40 and a letter (F, D, C, B, A). This corresponds to the University of Connecticut system of quality points and grades. (See figure 7-3 for Levels of Behavior and Point Values.)

At the inception of the curriculum, learners were advised that they had to earn a C- in each aspect of the nursing process in order to pass the clinical portion of the course. To comply with the university's grading policies, this decision was changed. The university policy indicates that a grade of D- is passing, so the original criteria for C- were moved down to D- and the interim levels of performance were redefined. The suggestion that this be done caused much debate. Some faculty felt that "D" behavior in professional practice would be unacceptable. This view is still held by many nurse educators, who continue to insist that "C" is the minimum grade for safe practice. People who believe this forget that the

A = EXCELLENT 40 Points	Displays indepth knowledge base Makes accurate judgments and recognizes conceptual relationships in complex situations Creatively applies principles to new practice situations
A- 37 Points	Displays self-direction in seeking valuable learning experiences Identifies strengths and weaknesses accurately
B+ 33 Points	
B = GOOD 30 Points	Displays above average knowledge base Makes accurate judgments and recognizes conceptual relationships Applies principles to practice setting
B- 27 Points	Self-directed and seeks guidance in searching out new learning experiences Identifies own strengths and weaknesses
C+ 23 Points	
C = AVERAGE 20 Points	Displays average knowledge base Accurate judgment; recognizes conceptual relationships with guidance Identifies principles that are applied in practice situations
C- 17 Points	Seeks learning experiences with guidance Identifies own strengths and weaknesses with guidance
D+ 13 Points	

D = POOR
10 Points
	Displays MINIMAL knowledge base
	Needs guidance to make accurate judgments and to recognize con-
	    ceptual relationships
	Uses safe technique in practice situations but cannot identify
	    supporting principles

D- 7 Points	Needs guidance to seek appropriate learning experiences Aware of strengths and weaknesses when identified by instructor

F = FAILING
0 Points
	Displays inadequate and/or unsafe knowledge base
	Makes inaccurate judgments and does not recognize conceptual re-
	    lationships
	Uses unsafe techniques in practice situations and is unable to
	    identify principles
	Does not make use of available learning experiences
	Unaware of strengths and weaknesses even when identified by in-
	    structor

FIGURE 7-3. Eighth semester process course, clinical laboratory grading guidelines, levels of behavior and point values.

letter is in itself meaningless. The important thing is that minimum acceptable performance be identified. This could be called X, Y, C, D or any other letter. It made sense to use the university grading system, however.

Determining Validity and Reliability

Determining the validity and reliability of the evaluative tools is the next step in the sequence of the evaluation process. This area of evaluation presents ongoing concerns and problems. As a measure of content validity, the faculty serves as a panel of experts and annually reviews and evaluates the content of the established criteria.

Reliability of the evaluation tools has not been documented. A suggestion is that faculty participate in inter-rater reliability activities. This could be accomplished by direct observation of the student or by the viewing of tapes of student performance by faculty. Individual faculty ratings could then be compared and a reliability coefficient computed. This suggestion has merit, but it was not given high priority and so has not yet been implemented.

Gathering Data

Gathering data is essential to the evaluation process. Supportive data for accomplishment of each objective from a variety of sources are provided by both learner and faculty. Student responsibility for documentation increases each semester of the program.

Faculty make direct observations of students in the clinical setting and record anecdotal notes. Students also submit such written assignments as nursing care plans, process recordings, and papers. Evaluative input from agency staff and clients is used when appropriate. Individual and group conferences provide another opportunity of gathering data for the evaluation process. The format of the clinical evaluation tool provides space next to each subobjective for making appropriate recordings of supportive evidence. An example is presented in figure 7-4.

Critically Interpreting Data

Critically interpreting data and assigning scores on the basis of outcomes is the fifth aspect of the evaluation process. The interpretatio

Objective	Points	Supportive Data
1.0 Design individualized nursing care plans for clients and/or families which reflect a focus on all actual and potential health problems.		
1.1 Collect a complete data base which reflects data from an assessment of the client, his family and/or significant others, and from previous or concurrent assessments conducted by other health team members.		*Health history complete* *Physical and developmental assessment accurate* *Compare with previous data and data collected by others*
1.2 Analyze the data to differentiate between normal and abnormal bio-psycho-social behaviors.		*Differentiates normal from abnormal* *Uses normal value scales* *Recognizes discrepancies*
1.3 After formulating a comprehensive problem list, deal with the problems according to priority.		*Sets priorities* *Combines problems that are related and/or conflicting*
1.4 Write behavioral objectives with specific outcome criteria for each problem in consultation with the client/family.		*Writes long and short term objectives, client centered, measurable* *Plans realistic goals* *Readjusts goals appropriately* *Evaluates outcome*
1.5 Identify nursing interventions which have a high probability for success in achieving the established outcome criteria.		*Identifies nursing intervention and alternatives* *Substantiates from literature* *Utilizes other health professionals as resources and plans with them*
1.6 Communicate the plan of care to all care providers.		*Uses Kardex* *Reports accurately during nursing conferences* *Appropriate written referrals and follow-up telephone calls*
Total Points	÷ 6 =	Section Average

FIGURE 7-4. Example of supportive data for one objective.

of data and scoring of laboratory activities are carried out by the learner and faculty advisor in individual and group conferences. Initially, the faculty advisor has major responsibility for completing the evaluation tools. The learner assumes increasing responsibility for his own evaluation as she progresses through the program. One aspect of Palmer's study (1959) explored self-evaluation. Palmer concluded that self-evaluation in determining grades was both reliable and valid based on correlations of .81 to .91 of instructor rating with student self-rating in two classes over a two-year period.

University of Connecticut faculty have also found that faculty and student ratings usually correlate quite well.

Evaluation takes place at predetermined times. Student and faculty advisor complete the evaluation tool independently. Then they review their findings in conference. Discussion follows on items where discrepancies are identified. In the rare instances where agreement cannot be reached, the faculty member makes the final decision.

Constructively Communicating the Results

Constructively communicating the results to those concerned completes the evaluation cycle. Faculty provide timely feedback informally throughout the semester as well as formally at least twice a semester. An important feature of the evaluation process is two-way communication. Learners are given the opportunity to make comments, raise questions, and seek clarification so that the experience is truly a learning situation. Preplanned evaluation conferences provide both the learner and faculty advisor with documentation of learner strengths and weaknesses. This documentation provides the basis for developing a plan to strengthen the desirable qualities and check undesirable behaviors. The students' professional growth is thus facilitated through the evaluation process. Crisis theory applied to student evaluation also strives to avert a crisis and, should one occur, to use it to foster student growth by developing appropriate coping mechanisms.

Outcomes of the Evaluative Process

The University of Connecticut faculty has addressed the difficult task of evaluating student achievement by stating a philosophy of evaluation and then operationalizing the philosophy through a systematic process. This has fostered the student's personal and professional growth and provided a basis for continuing self-evaluation as a graduate professional nurse. Furthermore, the student has learned principles and techniques of evaluation that can be applied to client care; health teaching of clients, families, and communities; and to peer review, which is becoming increasingly important in professional practice.

8

Issues and Problems

Linda R. Suess

A review of numerous articles that have been written about curriculum revision, as well as the earlier chapters of this book, make it clear that the process is never an easy one. It takes considerable time for faculty to express their anxieties, to work through feelings, and to analyze and discuss issues in order to reach consensus (Gordon & Anello, 1974; White & Coburn, 1977). Allowing time for the ventilation of feelings before pushing for task accomplishment may make the difference between success and failure of a curriculum project. If feelings are repressed and ignored they may fester and undermine the process. On the other hand, if open expression is encouraged and the behaviors associated with anxiety and grieving are understood and accepted, feelings and attitudes gradually change. Only then are faculty free to devote time and energy to the concrete tasks at hand.

The timetable for the University of Connecticut curriculum project allowed for several planning years prior to actual implementation. The innumerable planning meetings and informal discussions described in earlier chapters provided the vehicle for working through attitudes engendered by change and the threat of change. This was probably one reason the faculty was able, finally, to work effectively together and create and implement a well-conceived curriculum design.

Another positive factor was that certain individuals were able to exert effective leadership at crucial times. As a result, decisions were usually not finalized until the issues had been discussed from many points of view. Probing questions were asked in order to focus on the long-range implications of alternative solutions. If some individuals needed more time to ponder an issue and seek clarification before voting on a decision or making a commitment, this need was met. Many faculty often felt frustrated by the slowness of this decision-making process but, judging from the results, it proved to be worthwhile. The few decisions that were made without allowing sufficient time usually had to be reconsidered at a later date, thereby providing evidence that time coupled with patience is one key to success.

Another key factor was the willingness to take carefully considered risks, for major change is never without risk. For example, the fear that an integrated curriculum will not prepare students for State Board Examination nor for practice in a medically-oriented health care delivery system is not a groundless one. Lastly, it is important that individuals in leadership positions be prepared for faculty and student reaction to change as well as the problems inherent in an integrated curriculum. Then they may be viewed as factors that can be dealt with rather than as a signal to discard the new ideas and return to a more comfortable traditional approach to nursing content. The present chapter was written for this reason.

The focus of this chapter will be on problem areas most commonly identified by other schools (Bruton, 1974; Moloney, 1978; White & Coburn, 1977; Wolf-Wilets & Nugent, 1979; Styles, 1976; Murdock, 1978) as well as some that may be unique to the University of Connecticut. These problems have been categorized and discussed as follows: adjustment to team teaching; restructuring and reconceptualizing content; adapting teaching strategies; the generalist versus specialist role for faculty; implementing the philosophy of laboratory; and student reactions and problems.

IMPLEMENTING THE CURRICULUM DESIGN

Adjustment to Team Teaching

Chapter 5 has described the reorganization of faculty into two rather large teams, one for each level, with each team composed of faculty with diverse clinical backgrounds. This change provided a sharp contrast to the small homogeneous specialty teams that had characterized the former curriculum. Faculty were therefore anxious about their individual team assignments and about the appointment of team leaders (coordinators). Since the success of team functioning depends upon the establishment of trust among members and a successful blending of membership and leadership roles, a satisfactory early resolution of these two concerns was of paramount importance.

The assignment problem was resolved in a pragmatic way. Each faculty member completed a questionnaire stating her level preference (junior or senior) and a course preference (theory or process). In addition, the associate dean held many individual faculty conferences to discuss team assignments. Because faculty were given an opportunity to express preferences and make a choice, the end result was that the team assignments were acceptable to everyone. This laid the groundwork for the development of trust and relieved one source of anxiety.

The second concern was the selection of the coordinator. It was essential that this leader be someone who could do the following: inspire trust; foster healthy group process; encourage each individual to participate in discussions and decision making; recognize the reasons for various types of behavior and deal with them constructively; allow time for expression of ideas and questioning; and keep the group moving steadily toward task accomplishment.

The faculty had strong feelings about this position. A leader imposed by the administration without faculty input would probably not have secured the trust and cooperation needed during this very crucial period. On the other hand, it would have been unwise to base the decision completely on a faculty vote since factors other than competence might enter into the choice.

Securing a coordinator from outside the university who had not been involved with designing the curriculum and had thus not yet formed a commitment to it and who had no understanding of the internal politics might have been disastrous at that time. Therefore, the issue was resolved by selecting the coordinators from the current faculty. The selection process involved the team members and the dean. Each team was instructed to select three individuals that every team member was willing to support. The dean named the coordinator from among those three. This procedure continued satisfactorily until the organization structure of the school was changed in 1982.

With the resolution of the issues of membership and leadership, the newly-formed teams began to address the unfinished tasks. The quantity of work to be completed between May 30th and the implementation of fifth semester courses on September 1st created inevitable anxiety for the junior level team. These time constraints meant that the team did not have the luxury of working through the group process or of establishing trust among members and with the leader before implementing the newly-designed courses. However, by the end of the year, the team had reached a productive and cohesive level of functioning.

One issue that had to be resolved was that of individual autonomy versus group dependence. Faculty members could not work in isolation and make independent decisions that would affect the entire team. The team as a whole is responsible for the implementation of the curriculum and all parts have to fit together. In this type of teaching, many of the problems of planning and implementation are common to all team members. Therefore, frequent team meetings were necessary, especially in the beginning, to resolve problems and reach decisions. The best decisions were made when all members contributed their ideas and then, either through calm discussion or heated debate, a consensus was reached on the plan to be adopted. This consensus included identification of those areas that allow for individual differences and creativity.

Although frequent team meetings are probably unavoidable when a program is new and still evolving, the inordinate amount of time required may become burdensome and the concept of team teaching may thus be abandoned. One key to the success of large team functioning is to discriminate between issues that must be debated by the entire group and those which can be dealt with by a smaller task force or by one individual (Murdock, 1978). Issues that affect the entire team must be considered by that entire team. Problems that are more individual, such as the selection of clinical agencies for a particular group, can be decided by the individual faculty member or in collaboration with the coordinator.

As time progressed and faculty became more comfortable with the curriculum and with each other, they became more adept at discerning which issues could and could not be resolved without team consent and in facilitating the process of group decision making. To a large extent the problems of "ponderous teams" as described by Styles (1976) were resolved. More and more work is now completed by small task groups. This division of labor saves considerable time, minimizing the frequency and the length of team meetings. Relatively finished products are brought to the total team for approval. As a result, much less time is spent haggling over details and more time is available for substantive discussions that improve the quality of the program.

Another important factor in promoting team functioning is provision for feedback. At each team meeting, time is set aside to review major happenings and to identify the focus for classes and clinical activities. Individuals are also encouraged to share the methods they have used for meeting course objectives, especially those related to clinical laboratory. This includes both successes and failures. In this way the collective wisdom of the team can be used to devise more effective teaching strategies and also to facilitate correlation between the classroom and the clinical setting.

Another type of feedback relates to student (or graduate) achievement, particularly in the clinical setting. For example, comments from agency personnel, both solicited and unsolicited, are reported to the team. Positive comments bolster the morale and inspire even greater achievment: valid negative comments may form the basis for repairing a curriculum defect. Other aspects of team functioning will be considered under "Restructuring and Reconceptualizing Content" and "Implemting the Philosophy of Laboratory."

Restructuring and Reconceptualizing Content

"Unifying the nursing curriculum by means of the integrated approach means blending the nursing content in such a way that the parts or specialties are no longer distinguishable" (Torres, 1974, p. 2). This loss of a specialty focus generated problems for faculty whose education had prepared them as specialists. It was difficult to move from the traditional design, in which an entire course was devoted to each major clinical specialty, to one that reorganized content and scattered the familiar specialty subject among several courses. Faculty had to compete for time to teach their favorite subjects with the favorite subjects of their team members. They feared their specialty area would be covered superficially or lost altogether. It was equally threatening to be asked to teach unfamiliar content or to share the teaching of a favorite subject with a colleague in order to foster integration of concepts.

Allaying these fears and resolving these conflicts depended on learning to reconceptualize, to concentrate on generalizations relating to nursing rather than the specifics (Torres, 1974, p. 2), and to identify essential concepts. For faculty who had previously taught with a conceptual approach, the task was relatively easy. Others needed considerable help from colleagues. Faculty from different specialty areas met frequently to discuss common content. For example, the concept of pain crosses many areas, including pain associated with labor and delivery, injections in a child, surgery in an adult, and psychogenic pain with mental illness. Working through each concept to cover all aspects was difficult and challenging, but feasible. It did, of course, require compromises and the relinquishing of some cherished ideals (Wolf-Willets & Nugent, 1979).

One of the first attempts at integration in nursing involved inclusion of subjects such as pharmacology, pathobiology, and nutrition within nursing courses. Once the term "integration" had taken on a new meaning, the tendency was to delete non-nursing content. Faculty who formally included much pathobiology and pharmacology content in their classes now struggled with the task of defining nursing content and applying rather than teaching the content now included in other courses. The temptation to merely reteach the familiar material was great, and students were quick to notice and complain about any redundancy.

Any behavioral change of the magnitude just described takes time and energy. However, faculty worked through this painful process successfully. They audited each others' classes and provided feedback regarding the conceptualization of the content. This not only resulted in improved classes, but also in the development of a specific peer evaluation form that is used constantly and stimulates healthy dialogue before and after classes.

Utilization of crisis theory created problems for nearly all of the faculty. Not only did they need to delete pathobiology and pharmacology content and reconceptualize nursing content, they also had to put content into the crisis theory framework. Moloney's survey (1978) showed the problem of conceptualizing and organizing knowledge into a new framework to be a difficult task in many schools. In this instance, faculty with background in psychiatric nursing were essentially the only ones familiar with the concepts and terminology; all others had to learn crisis theory.

The process of learning and subsequently utilizing crisis theory was a threat as well as a challenge. Some faculty confronted the task immediately, while others waited until the last possible minute. Faculty familiar with the theory used it effectively and served as role models and mentors to those who struggled to learn it. The faculty shared literature that described the theory, met in many informal sessions to discuss use of the theory in the nursing courses, and provided critiques for each others' classes. The auditing of each others' classes insured the inclusion of essential content as well as improving the utilization of the crisis model.

Many faculty of different backgrounds now team teach particular classes to foster the concept of integrated learnings. The actual teaching is preceded by planning sessions and followed by an evaluation meeting. This has worked well, not only in providing in-depth education, but also in fostering communication and trust among team members. It has also reinforced the students' perception of nursing as a process.

Adapting Teaching Strategies

An additional problem that caused concern was how to teach large classes effectively. In the former curriculum pattern each total class was subdivided into several small sections that alternated through various nursing courses. Enrollment in a course averaged approximately 30-40 students. With the new curriculum design, an entire class takes all nursing courses together. This is necessary because of the carefully planned learning sequence described in Chapter 6. The result is a class enrollment of approximately 125 students.

Many hours were spent pondering teaching methods. Multiple strategies were identified that could be used with large groups. Some faculty had worked primarily with the lecture/discussion methods and felt most comfortable with these, while others preferred not to lecture. DeTornyay's work with various teaching strategies provided much needed information for dealing creatively with this problem (DeTornyay, 1971).

Faculty agreed that the most plausible answer was for each individual to use the methodology that was most comfortable for her and most appropriate to the content. Because of class size, the faculty initially tended to lecture with some discussion. As they became more comfortable with large groups, with the integrated concepts and content, and with the crisis framework, they tried new strategies. In fact, many strategies are now used, and the mixture is very conducive to learning. With some content it has been appropriate to divide the total class into small groups for discussion. This is particularly true for topics that are emotional or controversial, such as death and dying or abortion. This format is used frequently in the eighth semester when active student involvement is essential to the achievement of course objectives; at other times, role playing or case study presentations are effective.

In this way, the issue of the choice of teaching strategy has been resolved. Because content is dictated by the grid, faculty initially thought there would be no room left for individuality and creativity. It is now understood that while the general content is fixed, the teacher for each particular class has the freedom and the responsibility not only to determine specifics but also to select the teaching method most comfortable for her and most appropriate to the topic.

IMPLEMENTING THE LABORATORY COMPONENT

As difficult as designing an integrated curriculum is the task of implementing that design in clinical settings. One problem experienced by the University of Connecticut nursing faculty, as well as faculty in other schools (Moloney, 1978), is the expectation of teaching in a setting outside one's area of expertise. This can be termed the generalist versus specialist faculty role. A second problem is ensuring that no essential experiences are lost. Minimum requirements are mandated by state statute and also by professional expectations. The third problem—implementing the philosophy of laboratory—may in itself be unique to the University of Connecticut, but drives home an essential lesson of curriculum redesign. Each of these problem areas will be discussed.

Generalist/Specialist Role for Faculty

Styles has challenged the concept of integration by asking who or what exactly integrates whom or what (Styles, 1976). This question is basic to resolution of the issue of a generalist or specialist role for faculty. Faculty who believe it is the student who integrates may argue that faculty need not be generalists. If students and faculty both integrate, then the generalist role is an appropriate way to demonstrate this integration.

As the University of Connecticut curriculum was evolving, faculty assumed they would be expected to function as generalists, thereby relinquishing their specialist orientation. In fact, one source of anxiety was this threatened loss of identity with the clinical specialty for which they were prepared. In order to cope with change in orientation, faculty first needed to accept the concept of integrated learning experiences as valuable for students as well as feasible for themselves. Then preparation for the new role could begin.

When the curriculum design at the University of Connecticut was completed, it was obvious that, in a given semester, students would participate in a variety of clinical experiencs in many practice settings. Since each group of students was to remain with the same faculty advisor for an entire semester or a full year, faculty who were trying to function as generalists had to be prepared to practice and provide guidance in these various settings. This created problems and anxiety over the need to relearn skills related to unfamiliar practice settings. For example, a faculty member whose clinical expertise was in medical-surgical nursing might be guiding students in doing postpartum or newborn assessments. An individual prepared in psychiatric nursing might be guiding students doing colostomy care. This situation created a problem that required a carefully considered solution.

In order to reduce the threat to faculty as well as provide students with competent guidance, faculty utilized some unique approaches. Some informal classes were taught by faculty to their peers on such specific skills as newborn assessment. Other faculty requested experts to come to their agencies to help with student guidance in certain skills and reciprocated with their own areas of expertise. Some faculty developed videotapes on skills for use by students and faculty alike. Informal faculty discussions were held on various aspects of patient care. The faculty gradually became comfortable and competent in the new settings and needed less support from colleagues.

Several patterns for providing clinical guidance emerged. One of the factors that eased the transition from specialist to generalist was the formation of clinical regions with the built-in support systems described in Chapter 5. This facilitated the sharing of expertise described above. It also permitted establishment of a buddy system in which faculty remained in their area of expertise and students alternated between the areas. For example, a faculty expert in maternal-child nursing may team up with a medical-surgical expert. Students move from one faculty member to another. In this way faculty can provide expert assistance to students while they are together as well as facilitate the students' getting all appropriate experiences. Each faculty member also tries to incorporate additional concepts into his work with students. For example, a maternal-child nursing faculty member might challenge the student to consider care for a pregnant woman who has gallbladder disease, or a medical-surgical faculty member might challenge the student to imagine how care might be different for a patient with a fractured femur in skeletal traction if that patient were pregnant. This solution has worked very well in a number of regions.

In other regions, faculty developed a system whereby students spend some time with each of the faculty specialists but have one major advisor who is responsible for planning learning experiences with her, guiding the Family Study, and evaluating achievement. In addition, some faculty chose to function as generalists immediately, guiding their students in all clinical areas.

Student response to the various patterns of clinical teaching have been supportive to all of them. Some prefer the generalist teacher, while others prefer exposure to several generalists/specialists during a year. All patterns have resulted in satisfactory student achievement of course objectives.

It is essential that faculty be allowed to resolve the problem of clinical role, with its inherent anxiety, in creative ways. Not all individuals are capable of working out problems in the same manner. All of the solutions have worked well and they have significantly reduced the threat of working in unfamiliar clinical settings with unfamiliar skills. This acceptance of individual differences among faculty has been important to the success of the curriculum. No attempt has been made to require a faculty member to do something for which she feels utterly unprepared. However, each faculty member has agreed to set learning goals for herself and to gradually expand her sphere of functioning. It should be noted that the number of faculty choosing to function as generalists has increased markedly during the eight years the curriculum has been operational. The issue is still being debated, however, perhaps because there are no indisputable data to either support or reject the generalist posture for faculty in an integrated curriculum. More research is needed on this important issue to provide substantive data to support one approach or another.

Perhaps the nature of graduate education itself is at the root of the controversy. Until recently, graduate education has produced specialists—a factor that may support feelings of distress when faculty encounter the generalist role in the integrated curriculum (Moloney, 1978). If undergraduate integrated curricula are here to stay, changes in graduate programs are needed. The curriculum described in Chapter 10 is a sound step in that direction.

From the discussion presented thus far, it is apparent that faculty had many learning needs when this new curriculum was being implemented. They had to learn new relationships, new teaching methods, a different way of conceptualizing, and also to relearn skills related to unfamiliar clinical settings. In addition, they had to learn physical assessment theory and skills. The curriculum design included this content in the first semester of the junior year, and few faculty had a solid knowledge base in this area. The principle that "learning is most effective when an individual is ready to learn, that is, when he feels a need to know something" (Redman, 1972, p. 40), was certainly applicable to the learning needs of the faculty at the time. Fortunately, one faculty member was well prepared in physical assessment and was assigned to teach her colleagues. It was not difficult for faculty to learn the theory, but learning the psychomotor skills was time-consuming and often anxiety-provoking.

One problem associated with learning physical assessment skills was timing. According to the grid, students begin to learn physical assessment in the fifth semester process course. At the time this course was first implemented, faculty were just beginning to learn the basic elements of assessment. In fact, they taught this content only a few days after learning it themselves. This meant that they were merely a step ahead of the students and felt uncomfortable and insecure. This was not educationally sound, although probably unavoidable. The pressure of curriculum development had left no time or energy for an earlier inservice program in physical assessment.

Essential Clinical Learnings

The change from a traditional curriculum to an integrated one created yet another problem—the need to identify the clinical learnings that were essential for all students. A traditional curriculum generally has nursing courses related to a particular practice specialty, such as psychiatric or pediatric nursing. Such courses last either a partial semester or an entire one. Within these courses, there is usually ample time for students to complete a wide variety of learning experiences related to that specialty area.

An integrated curriculum does not have as much time inherent in its design. In fact, such a specialty approach is contrary to the very definitions of conceptual and integrative learnings. Yet, the state requirements for practice are still defined in terms of the traditional clinical specialties. It thus becomes imperative to define which clinical learnings preserve the integrity of the framework, reflect course objectives, concepts, and content, and assure a well-rounded experiential background appropriate for beginning practice.

Initially, faculty provided what appeared to be appropriate experiences for their respective groups of students. While absolutely identical experiences were neither possible nor desirable, there was concern about the limited uniformity between clinical groups. Another concern of school administrators was the need to demonstrate compliance with State Board of Nursing requirements.

The initial impetus for studying this problem came from faculty members who were prepared in community health. They expressed a strong concern that community health content and concepts were underrepresented in this new curriculum design. In order to see if this was, in fact, true, these faculty met to review what was included in the curriculum, what additional content and/or experience was needed, and what were the essential clinical learnings within the scope of community health practice.

As a result of this initial work, faculty from other specialties also met to identify essential learnings within their respective areas (Murdock, 1978). Lengthy lists of essential learnings were produced that necessitated debate and negotiation to achieve a complete yet feasible level of requirements. The outcome was the development of clinical models representing major concepts with a variety of suggested as well as required activities. For example, within the well-child model, each student must perform a faculty-precepted Denver Developmental Screening Test. This may be done in any setting where there is a child of testable age. Students identify the normal growth and development patterns of well children; they may do this in schools, day-care centers, clinics, or physicians' offices. This allows some flexibility in how one meets the required objective.

Both the junior and senior levels developed models reflecting specific content and practice areas and providing guidelines for selection of clinical activities. The first draft of essential clinical learnings was used on a trial basis and then revised. The clinical models have been replaced with a format consistent with the conceptual framework, and more descriptive guidelines have been formulated. This system works well. It provides for well-balanced learning experiences and identifies specifically how students meet state requirements for practice. Students keep records that help both faculty and students to visualize the student's progress in meeting the course objectives and the directions in which further work is desirable or essential. The junior level experience record is given to the student's senior level advisor to be used as a basis for planning learning needs for the senior year.

Implementing the Philosophy of Laboratory

In Chapter 7, the philosophy of laboratory, written by faculty in order to provide guidance for the laboratory aspects of the nursing courses, was described. All faculty had input into this document and it appeared to be reflective of the faculty's beliefs. However, actual use of the philosophy created problems in both college and clinical laboratory.

During the first year of the new program, policies relating to the college laboratory reflected faculty belief that students should be independent, self-paced learners. Therefore, at the beginning of the semester, students were given a list of required laboratory activities with no specific due dates except the end of the semester. This proved to be somewhat analogous to throwing a child in the water for the first time telling him to swim, although faculty did not notice immediately that students were drowning. It was not until mid-semester that faculty realized how few students had even begun to meet the course requirements for college laboratory activities.

Analysis of the problem revealed that faculty who were teaching about developmental levels and needs had neglected to assess the students' developmental levels. Up to this time, students had been educated in a structured system where little independence was encouraged. As late adolescents, they still needed some direction in setting their own limits. Faced with total independence, they reacted with immobility. The solution was a system of establishing due dates at intervals throughout the semester, as described in Chapter 7. Students can, however, pace themselves in their reading, viewing of media, and practicing in the laboratory. They like this arrangement—it gives them appropriate responsibility for their learning and supports the Rogerian belief that "learning is facilitated when the student participates responsibly in the learning process" (Rogers, 1969, p. 162).

The issue of student independence has also affected the staffing of the college laboratory. Many faculty believe that the intended use of the college laboratory mandates that students practice independently and then be evaluated by laboratory staff with very little input from staff. Other faculty members believe that students need feedback and guidance during practice sessions in order to enhance learning; otherwise time is wasted, and students become frustrated. Also, some see the laboratory as a place for creative teaching strategies, not just independent student learning.

Beliefs about the use of the college laboratory have implications for the number and qualifications of laboratory staff. The issue is still unresolved. The questions to be answered are: Should the laboratory be staffed by baccalaureate-prepared nurses who manage logistics, monitor practice, and evaluate achievement according to faculty developed critical elements? Or is this laboratory an integral part of the process course and a place where teaching strategies are planned and implemented by qualified faculty? In order to resolve the issue, research is needed to test out various methods, including the theories related to psychomotor skill learning presented in Chapter 7.

The most emotionally charged aspect of the philosophy of laboratory in its original form was the part relating to clinical laboratory Some faculty believed it should be interpreted strictly. Others felt there was room for a liberal interpretation. Still others were not quite sure how to interpret it. Almost everyone had misconceptions about what it actually said. This confusion led to difficulties in explaining the philosophy to students and agency staff as well as in implementing it.

All these difficulties were the result of a more basic problem—the philosophy did not accurately reflect faculty beliefs. It had been written during the period when faculty were concentrating on completing the curriculum design and developing outlines for courses. While there were strong feelings about laboratory, the philosophy had not been discussed openly at great length before being accepted.

The major turning point was a well-timed consultation visit. Having read the philosophy, the consultant questioned the intent of several sections. With relief that the issue of the philosophy was finally out in the open, much discussion ensued. Difficulties of interpretation and implementation were shared. The end result of this discussion was a review and editing of the document to more accurately reflect faculty beliefs.

In retrospect, many of the problems associated with the philo phy probably resulted from insufficient discussion and the conse- quent misunderstanding of issues. The problems have been described here in order to emphasize the importance of thorough discussion as the groundwork for understanding and consistent implementation of each aspect of a new curriculum.

It is essential for faculty to develop a philosophy of laboratory prior to a curriculum's actual implementation. If, however, an innovative and/or potentially controversial statement is being drafted, it would be prudent to provide faculty with needed time and, ideally, an objective consultant to openly discuss implementation. Some authors have suggested that any statement of philosophy be kept in rough form until the curriculum is completed (Gordon & Anello, 1974). Periodic review can identify problems and establish needed changes that more accurately reflect philosophic beliefs, thereby avoiding unnecessary distress. This did happen with the philosophy of the program, which was internalized without the up- heaval associated with the philosophy of laboratory.

STUDENT REACTIONS AND PROBLEMS

The last section of this chapter deals with student reactions and some special student problems related to the implementation of this new, integrated curriculum. Students responded in a variety of ways. Their reactions were similar to those of the faculty and ran the gamut from excitement to a high level of anxiety and even hos- tility. When faculty felt doubtful and anxious, students would sense these feelings and react similarly. As faculty doubts changed to excitement and faith in the program, so did student response.

Students in the first class exhibited behaviors consistent with the "First Class Syndrome." They felt they were guinea pigs in an experimental program—these reactions expanded into fears that the program would not prepare them adequately for professional prac- tice. Their parents also expressed concern regarding the credi- bility of this new program (White & Coburn, 1977).

The rumor mill was very active and circulated many messages that served to heighten already high anxiety levels. It was rumored that the school would lose its accreditation; that the nursing courses were mainly theoretical, with little clinical experience; that the school functioned with a quota system and that attempts would be

t" numbers of students before they reached the
ler to reduce class size. The chemistry courses
he ones that would decide who would stay and who
ist rumor heightened anxiety as well as the compe-
igh grades in order to be among the few who would

scribed the planned orientations for new curricu-
lum students, including class meetings as well as small group and
one-to-one conferences to answer questions and quell rumors. A
student handbook was also developed that described the student-
faculty advisory system and provided easy access to information
about the program. During the first few years, however, when some
courses had not yet been taught, the answers students were looking
for were not yet available. This also heightened anxiety. Students
were able to tolerate this uncertainty when faculty listened to their
concerns, quelled rumors, and gave honest answers, even if the
answers were necessarily vague. When the faculty appeared to have
faith and confidence, those feelings were transmitted to students.
The reverse, of course, was also true.

Students faced an unexpected problem when they began their
clinical experiences. Many agencies had participated in the former
nursing curriculum and were familiar with the focus and requirements of the courses. With implementation of the new curriculum,
agency staff bombarded students with questions about the program,
and shared with these students their doubts and concerns regarding
its adequacy. Students found themselves in the awkward position of
describing their program to agency staff, and, in many instances,
having to defend its quality. Initially, faculty had to help students
who were still doubtful to deal with this unanticipated situation. However, students in the first class, as well as subsequent classes,
soon became articulate in explaining and defending the program.

Faculty had been prepared for the reactions of students in the
new program, but they had not been prepared for the hostility expressed by the senior class in the outgoing curriculum. Students in
the last class reacted strongly to the curriculum change. Initially,
their feelings were similar to those of students in the new program.
They were thus very thankful that they were a part of the old program. In fact, they heightened the anxiety of new students by cor-
roborating their fears. These warnings included the lower division
courses, which the seniors agreed had been selected to enhance the
weeding-out process and would be nearly impossible to pass.

As the time for actual implementation of the new upper divi: grew near, the reaction of this last class began to change. Dur... their senior year, as they witnessed the implementation of the junior year of the new curriculum, this change in attitude became apparent. Their response changed to a feeling of being cheated. They became interested in the new conceptual approach and were envious of the inclusion of physical assessment skills in the new program. Students became concerned that something must have been wrong with their curriculum to warrant such complete revision, and they worried that they were not adequately prepared for practice.

Faculty endeavored to assist the senior students to deal with their anger. They were assured that their program had prepared them for current practice, and that the success of previous graduates proved that. Frequent class meetings allowed students to ventilate their concerns and to receive current information on different aspects of the program. Faculty advisors made a special effort to enrich their senior experiences and meet individual needs. In some instances, selected parts of physical assessment were taught to the senior students. They also discussed the different curriculum approaches in nursing education in order to prepare them for a changing health care system. At the time of graduation, most of the seniors agreed they had had an enriching year and felt proud of themselves and of their curriculum.

Now that the integrated program has been functioning effectively for several years, the focus of student reaction has changed. Instead of worrying about the quality of the program, students worry about themselves. Whether they will succeed or not has become the focus of their anxiety. The faculty has been able to foster positive attitudes with the help of articulate students. A few seniors attend a junior class, and both seniors and juniors attend freshman and sophomore class meetings to explain what the program is like and to tell them that they will make it if they study hard. Honest responses to concerns and issues have fostered trust in the quality of the program and in the students themselves. Students enjoy learning of the activities of upperclassmen and also of graduates, and, whenever possible, talking with these people directly.

One other type of student problem, associated with the curriculum design described in this book, deserves mentioning. It is not a problem for those students, still in the majority, who follow the prescribed pattern and complete the program in four years. However, there seems to be an increasing number of so-called exceptional students—students who drop out temporarily for financial, health, or other personal reasons. Also, some students are electing to carry a lighter load to permit time to work or cope with family responsibilities or because of academic problems. Moreover, a few students might be capable of accelerating, but they are all handicapped by the lock-step nature of the curriculum.

Because each nursing semester builds on the previous one, the sequence of courses cannot be changed. Neither can the nursing sequence proceed without completing the prerequisite general education and supportive courses. This pattern is educationally sound. However, it means that missing one course may mean that a student loses an entire year because often courses are offered only once a year and not in summer school. Failing a required course in the upper division has the same result.

The curriculum would allow much more flexibility if courses were offered each semester and/or in summer school. However, a large enrollment in each course would be necessary to make it economically feasible for the school. A team taught course is particularly expensive if offered in summer school.

Integrated curricula also make it difficult for students to transfer from one baccalaureate nursing program to another. Even two integrated programs may have such a different approach and sequence that it is impossible to identify any transferable equivalents. In order to avoid serious gaps, the transfer student may have to start at the beginning of the nursing sequence although sometimes individualized programs can be developed to remedy deficits and reduce the time needed for completion.

Another exceptional student population is that group of registered nurses who have graduated from an associate degree or diploma nursing program and seek the baccalaureate degree in nursing. These students come from varied backgrounds, and require individually designed programs to meet their needs. Some students have earned credit for courses, while others have earned no acceptable college credits. In most instances, students lack the strong general education background required in this curriculum and must take nearly all of the required lower division courses.

Transfer credit is not given for nursing courses. Although the R.N. student is familiar with much of the basic content and the skills, the courses he/she has had are not comparable to those in the University of Connecticut program. Since it is not possible to obtain transfer credit for a part of a course and register for the other part, a different method of earning credit is needed.

Redman has described the quandary of trying to find a mutual fit with educational needs and past experiences for this group of exceptional students (Redman, 1974). One solution for dealing with the problem is to offer challenge examinations where the student can demonstrate his knowledge and skills. This does not eliminate the problem described above, since a student may successfully challenge aspects of the course but not be prepared to take an examination on an entire course. It is possible, however, for the R.N. to study independently and earn approximately half of the upper division nursing credits by examination, thereby completing the upper division in one year instead of the usual two years.

When a registered nurse does enroll in a nursing course, the faculty advisor assesses her learning needs and provides individualized experiences in order to capitalize on her strengths and remedy her deficits. This is particularly true when planning laboratory experiences. Students have responded positively to many of their experiences but the problem is still unresolved. As Styles has suggested, it may be advisable to develop a separate track for the R.N./B.S. student (Styles, 1976). Further investigation and research into this problem may result in a pattern of education that is a better fit for these students. The University of Connecticut has designed a research proposal to address these problems and has established a counseling center for graduate nurses seeking a degree.

A discussion of exceptional students is not complete without mentioning the University Honors Program for superior students. In this program, students may enroll in specific honors sections of courses or elect to receive honors credit within a normal course structure. Since there usually is not a large enough number of honors students in nursing to warrant a separate honors section in a nursing course, students must demonstrate honors work within the regular course structure. Although this sounds simple, it presents problems.

Part of the difficulty stems from philosophical differences of faculty. Some faculty believe that honors should not involve extra work, but added depth in required assignments, while others feel that honor students should study in addition to regular course requirements. Faculty also differ in their individual interpretation of what constitutes honors work. Some believe it should be research-oriented, while others feel that this expectation is unrealistic, especially at the junior level. As a result, honors work can be as varied as the individual faculty advisor's interpretation of it. Some faculty believe the educational needs of the superior student should be provided for, while others argue that it is difficult to provide enrichment when a student is unfamiliar with the basic components of nursing.

Many approaches have been used. A separate section of a nursing process course, designated as a seminar for honors students, worked well when the number of students was approximately 15. However, only two or three students in a class may be enrolled in the honors program at a time, so a separate section is not always feasible in terms of faculty time.

Honor students have been allowed to complete honors work in two other ways within the normal course structure: to complete additional requirements, or to contract for different requirements. As mentioned before, this has caused concern in the identification of what constitutes honors work and also in the actual grading process. The mechanics of deciding on the number of honors credits a particular project is worth has been difficult. One solution that has worked well has been to identify specific options within a course, with specific credit allotment and grading criteria identified.

Perhaps the easiest solution is that of having students earn honors credits through independent study courses. While this solution adds extra work to an already demanding course load, it gives students more freedom to propose projects and select an appropriate credit allocation while earning additional credits for graduation. An honors committee continues to study this problem and search for creative solutions.

SUMMARY

This chapter has described the major problems experienced and, for the most part, resolved by the University of Connecticut faculty during the process of designing and implementing a unique curriculum. While some may argue that the price to be paid in time and energy for a curriculum revision characterized by team teaching and the eradication of traditional clinical specialties exceeds normal capability, the University of Connecticut faculty believe that the rewards far outweigh the price. They enjoy built-in opportunities to discuss common issues in nursing that cross the clinical specialty areas. They have developed skill in conceptualizing and in dealing with content formerly outside their areas of expertise and they have, in fact, expanded those areas of expertise. A trusting relationship has been established among faculty members and between students and faculty.

Faculty have experienced the pleasure of observing students develop the ability to conceptualize, to transfer familiar concepts to unfamiliar situations, to internalize the crisis theory framework, and to use it successfully in their practice. They have observed with pride the accomplishments of the graduates of this program. The benefits gained by faculty in educational as well as in personal achievements have motivated them to accept new challenges in education, practice, and research.

9

Evaluating the Curriculum
Marguerite B. White

The systematic evaluation of educational endeavors has become a way of life. Just as no course outline is complete without a statement of methods for evaluating student achievement, no curriculum design is complete without a plan for evaluating its effectiveness. Chapter 7 has addressed the subject of student evaluation. This chapter will describe the curriculum evaluation plan, the problems of its implementation, and some of its findings. Evaluation theory will not be presented since that is beyond the scope of this book.

In 1967, Scriven first differentiated two roles for educational evaluation—summative and formative. The former evaluates the effectiveness of a program in terms of the end product—in this case, the graduate. Summative evaluations that compare two curricula assume that the programs remain basically unchanged during the data collection period. Formative evaluation provides for periodic data collection and feedback about segments of the curriculum or curriculum materials. It is used for ongoing evaluation and minor improvements that do not affect the integrity of the curriculum design. Both summative and formative evaluation methods are described in the following pages.

SUMMATIVE EVALUATION

The major purpose of the summative evaluation plan was to determine the effectiveness of the revised curriculum in educating a professional nurse. The plan involved a comparison between students and graduates of the revised curriculum and those of the traditional program. It included measurement of characteristics considered important for nursing as well as achievement. A second purpose was the collection of data that might be useful in revising policies regarding admission and progress of students.

In order to collect base line data for students in the outgoing curriculum as well as for entering students in the new program, decisions about criterion measures needed to be made when the envisioned curriculum was little more than a dream. However, a philosophy had been drafted and global program objectives developed. Using these materials and the National League for Nursing characteristics of baccalaureate education, the project director and an evaluation consultant identified behaviors that the curriculum would ideally achieve. Creativity, self-motivation, independence, and a view of professional nursing very different from the commonly held stereotype were some of the factors initially identified as desirable outcomes.

Instruments were selected or constructed to measure student abilities, values, personality factors, and perceptions. In addition, National League for Nursing tests in the four clinical areas—medical-surgical, maternal-child, psychiatric nursing, and community health—as well as the State Board examinations, were readily available standardized measures of achievement. Follow-up tools for graduates and their employers were designed to provide measures of the program's effectiveness in the professional world.

The testing schedule, which began with seniors in the class of 1971 and ended with the class of 1978, is presented in table 9-1. The Scholastic Aptitude Test scores, required of all entering freshmen at the university, were a readily available means of establishing a base line in terms of academic ability. Several of the criterion measures were administered three times to each class of students. Using old curriculum students as controls, it was hoped some conclusions could be reached about changes in personality characteristics, values, and creative ability that might be attributable to the new curriculum. In addition, the data were to be used to develop a prediction equation for performance in nursing by relating measures of attitude and personality to achievement.

The Strong Vocational Interest Blank, which was replaced in 1973 by the Strong Campbell Interest Inventory, was also selected for its potential predictive value. Factor analysis was to be used to construct a key that might help in identifying students with good

TABLE 9-1. The Evaluation Plan[*]

Variables to be Measured	Tools for Measurement	Timetable of Measurements
Student Abilities, Values, and Personality Factors	Scholastic Aptitude Test	Prior to admission
	Torrance Test of Creative Thinking[a]	Semesters 1, 4, 8
	Strong Vocational Interest Blank[a]	Semester 1
	Survey of Values[a]	Semesters 1, 4, 8
	California Psychological Inventory	Semesters 1, 4, 8
	Survey of Interpersonal Values[b]	Semesters 1, 4, 8
	Strong Campbell Interest Inventory[c]	Semester 1
Student Perceptions	Semantic Differential-Meanings of Professional Occupations Scale	Semesters 1, 4, 8
	Nursing School Environmental Inventory[d]	Semester 8
Graduate Perceptions	Follow-up Questionnaire	Post graduation 1 & 3 years
Student Achievement	National League for Nursing Achievement Tests	Semester 8
	Nursing State Board Examinations	Post graduation
Graduate Achievement	Follow-up Questionnaires: Ratings of Self Ratings of Employer Professional Achievements, Contributions, Growth	Post graduation 1 & 3 years

[*]Reprinted from Final Report of Five Year Curriculum Project, University of Connecticut School of Nursing, 1977.

[a]Dropped from the plan

[b]Added to the plan to replace the Survey of Values

[c]Added to the plan to replace the Strong Vocational Interest Blank, but not included in final analysis

[d]Added to the plan

potential for nursing. This use of data to predict success rather than as a measure of curriculum effectiveness is an example of an administrative question that may be answered through curriculum evaluation data.

The Semantic Differential-Meanings of Professional Occupations Scale was adapted from a tool designed for an evaluative study at the University of Connecticut School of Pharmacy. This questionnaire was designed to gather demographic data and to measure attitudes toward and perceptions of the role of the nurse and other health care professionals. It, too, was to be administered three times in order to detect changes that might be attributable to the curriculum.

The Nursing School Environmental Inventory was developed by Johnson in 1971 based on the Medical School Environmental Index constructed by Edwin Hutchins (Johnson, 1971). It measured the following student perception factors (University of Connecticut School of Nursing, 1974):

1. General esteem—general factor
2. Academic interest and enthusiasm—extent to which students seek academic excellence and faculty is enthusiastic about subject matter.
3. Extrinsic motivation—includes faculty strictness, close supervision of students, faculty pressure to achieve, emphasis on students avoiding clinical mistakes by working together.
4. Breadth of interest—extent to which faculty and students share interests outside of nursing.
5. Intrinsic motivation—extent to which environment does not pressure students and students behave and are treated as adults.
6. Encapsulated training—extent to which instruction is well-organized with little divergence from a prescribed curriculum

This tool was administered to seniors to solicit their perceptions of the learning environment in the School of Nursing.

Unquestionably, the true test of a curriculum's effectiveness is the competence and achievements of its graduates. Even though it is practically impossible to separate the effects of the educational program from postgraduate influences, no evaluation is complete without a follow-up study. As early as the first year of the project, efforts were directed toward the creation of a follow-up instrument.

It was relatively easy to develop a biographical questionnaire to elicit information about graduates' activities. Assessing knowledge and skills one and three years after graduation was not so simple. The first attempt, which consisted of a simulation exercise that was pretested on faculty, was such a total failure that a decision was made to await publication of the proposed National League for Nursing test modules and to adapt them for use in assessing graduates.

By spring 1975, the above-mentioned test modules were not yet available. Even if they had been, the practicality of adapting them to the intended purpose was questionable. The curriculum project committee therefore developed a tool using program objectives as a general guide.

In addition to biographical data, the questionnaire solicits the graduates' perceptions of the value of the curriculum and his or her self-evaluation as a practitioner. Questionnaires used by other universities for a similar purpose were reviewed. Particularly helpful were the tools developed by the University of Virginia School of Nursing (Taylor & Mandrillo, 1973) and by Marlene Kramer for the University of California School of Nursing graduates. Since the latter had been validated, it was adapted and used, with Kramer's permission, as the basis for the self-evaluation section of the instrument. Another source of ideas was Reality Shock by Marlene Kramer (1974).

A draft of the tool was tested by circulating it to faculty with a request for suggestions. Following this, appropriate revisions were made. A second instrument was developed to be administered to graduates' employers. This version requests that the employer rate the performance of the graduate and is an adaptation of the self-evaluation section of the first instrument. Items are identical except for changes in pronouns.

PROBLEMS AND FRUSTRATIONS

It has been said that the opportunity to be on hand at the initiation of a curriculum change and to collect and analyze data on all three phases of the process (inputs, thruputs, and outputs) is an evaluator's dream (Green & Stone, 1977). It can also be a nightmare. The frustrations attendant upon implementation of a seven-year plan are seemingly endless. Following are some examples.

Changes in Measurement Tools

Both the Study of Values and the Strong Vocational Interest Blank
were judged to be outdated after they had been administered to several classes. This posed a dilemma—should more valid instruments
be substituted, thereby eliminating some of the data, or should the
original plan be retained? The decision was made to replace the
outdated tests with the Survey of Interpersonal Values and the Strong-
Campbell Interest Inventory. Therefore, data for some earlier
classes were lost.

The Torrance Test of Creativity was another source of problems. It was very time-consuming to administer and costly to have
scored. All the other tests could be given to students in a packet to
take home; the Torrance Test of Creativity requires timed, moni-
tored administration, and student cooperation was poor. In addition
to these administrative problems, there is no evidence that the Torrance Test of Creativity actually measures the kind of creativity
needed in nursing. The use of this tool was therefore discontinued,
again leaving the project with useless data.

In 1973 the National League for Nursing substituted new tests
in Psychiatric Nursing and Community Health Nursing. This meant
that scores in these two subjects for the classes of 1971 and 1972
were useless for comparison purposes. In 1978 the Maternal-Child
test was changed, so that only two of the new curriculum classes
(1976 and 1977) can be compared with the old curriculum on that criterion measure.

In addition to the changes described above, two measures were
selected after the evaluation process had started. These are the
Semantic Differential Meaning of Professional Occupations Scale and
the Nursing School Environmental Inventory. Therefore, there is
little control data available for comparison between old and new curricula. However, it is possible to compare changes that occur in
new curriculum students during the four-year program.

Securing Student Cooperation

Another frustration for any evaluator is the problem of gaining student cooperation. There was a time in nursing's history when students would scarcely have dared to refuse to do what they were told,
for example, to appear at a designated time and place to complete a
questionnaire or test. But times have changed. Independence in

students, and even a bit of rebellion, are now valued and nurtured. Moreover, societal changes have placed high priority on students' rights. A school cannot legally require participation in any activity that is not a requirement for graduation and so stated in the university catalogue.

Since participation in data collection was voluntary, the evaluators tried various methods for securing student cooperation. Success was less than hoped for with old curriculum students. Project staff naively thought that new curriculum students would cooperate at a high percentage because they would be imbued with the concepts of professional responsibility and commitment and convinced of the value of participating in research. This did not prove to be true. The evaluators tried personal letters, class announcements, and posters on bulletin boards. They appealed to students' altruism and professional responsibility. They scheduled alternative testing dates and places and also pointed out to students the personal value of knowing their own scores. They stressed that participation was a school expectation even if not an absolute requirement. They even resorted to paying non-nursing control subjects. Results were disappointing.

Administering tests during a regular class period or as an assignment for a psychology course proved somewhat successful. The best results were achieved when, in 1975, the procedure of administering all tests through a take-home packet was instituted. Obviously, National League for Nursing achievement tests could not be administered in this way. However, emphasizing the value of these examinations as preparation for State Board Examinations was quite successful. Unfortunately, there is no State Board Examination in Community Health Nursing, which probably accounts for the smaller number of students taking that test.

As early as the second year of the project, the evaluation plan included testing of non-nursing University of Connecticut students in order to differentiate between changes or differences that might be due to maturation or to university factors rather than to the curriculum. The experience with controls corroborates the following comment by Greene and Stone, "In curriculum projects, the classic design of comparison groups often turns sour because equivalent groups are not practical, or worse yet . . . in time the control group simply fades away entirely or becomes too small for statistical comparison" (1977, p. 31). After three years of struggling, the efforts to find non-nursing control subjects was discontinued, and many of the subjects recruited early in the project did indeed fade away. In fact, the data collected from this group are not sufficient enough to be meaningful.

Missing or Noncomparable Data

It is obvious from the foregoing discussion that data are missing because some measures were added or changed after the data collection had started. It is equally obvious that because of lack of cooperation for all criterion measures except the State Board examinations, the data are on a nonrandom sample of students rather than the total population. For some subjects the data base is nearly complete and for others there are many missing data because the students did not participate in every aspect of the testing program.

Another complicating factor in any longitudinal study of college students that seeks to compare one class with another is that class membership does not remain stable. For a variety of reasons, students transfer in and out of programs at various points. Some take time off or decide to proceed more slowly, thereby dropping back a year or two, and some do not complete the program at all. Some of these problems were solved by developing a formula for defining class membership. At times there was no solution except to discard the data.

Miscellaneous Sources of Frustration or Invalid Data

It is probably impossible for two different curricula to proceed side by side and not influence each other. This has been pointed out by other evaluators (for example, Green & Stone, 1977). Chapter 8 describes some of the feelings and anxieties that the curriculum change engendered in both old and new curriculum students and also in faculty. These feelings had an unavoidable effect on the outcomes of both programs and the subjects' responses to the criterion measures.

As pointed out earlier, changes take place as a program is evolving, based on formative evaluation. One would therefore expect the curriculum to become increasingly strong and the students to achieve at a higher level on standardized tests. Interestingly, the situation was reversed. The first class in the new curriculum had a very small failure rate, only three percent, on the State Board Examinations. With successive classes, this leveled off to a more usual rate even though the content of courses had been strengthened. The success of the first class may be attributed partly to a Hawthorne effect and partly to greater academic ability as evidenced by higher verbal SAT scores.

CONCLUSIONS

What can be learned from the University of Connecticut experiences? There are no guaranteed solutions to the problems described on the preceding pages, but an awareness of the potential pitfalls may make it easier to avoid them. For example, when the follow-up tool was drafted, the focus of the evaluation design was a comparison of the outcomes of the two curricula. Therefore, it seemed appropriate to include only items that were relevant to graduates of both programs. In 1977, after sending the questionnaire to the first of the new curriculum graduates, a serious omission was noted—no items addressed the crisis theory model. Faculty were anxious to know to what extent graduates were using the model in their practice, but that information was not available: a page was added to the questionnaire to be sent to subsequent classes.

Perhaps the need to make changes in the evaluation plan was unavoidable since it had been initiated so early in the curriculum development process; if so, the disadvantages of this early beginning should be accepted along with the advantages. A sound suggestion would be to take care in selecting or developing instruments to be sure that they measure that which is really important to measure. Also, care should be taken that they not become outdated before the project is finished. This may minimize the amount of useless or unusable data.

Secondly, the number of tests or questionnaires students are asked to complete should be kept to a minimum. Student cooperation will be better if demands are fewer; greater participation was secured with take-home test packets than with group testing on specified dates. Lastly, if students can be convinced that their participation is of personal value, their motivation is apparently higher. Obviously, using ready-made data such as Scholastic Aptitude Test scores and State Board Examination scores is the surest way of obtaining maximum participation.

FORMATIVE EVALUATION

The discussion has thus far described the summative or end product evaluation. Equally as important and as time-consuming is the on-going or formative evaluation that provides frequent feedback and is used to modify aspects of the program before summative data are available. Decisions regarding the utilization of this type of data involve some philosophical issues. For example, how much change is permissible? Faculty had agreed that no substantive changes would be made until three years after the termination of the project. That time period would make possible the initiation of carefully considered change based on summative data.

What constitutes a substantive change? Common sense provides the best answer. For example, if faculty experts in maternal-child nursing believe that the courses include insufficient content in their area of specialization and National League for Nursing and State Board Examination scores in this area are low, it would make sense to strengthen the content in that area and search for more effective learning experiences. Such a change can be made without changing the curriculum design or the conceptual model.

This example raises another question—who has the authority to make such changes and what are the mechanisms for change? A general policy adopted by the University of Connecticut was that any change affecting the total program must be approved by the total faculty. Less significant changes could be made by the teaching team. The grid depicting course content includes major concepts to be taught at each level. These were developed from the conceptual framework and are expected to remain basically unchanged. However, there is considerable latitude for altering details of content and changing the emphasis in order to improve effectiveness and also to keep up to date and relevant.

To give another example, junior level faculty do not have the freedom to ignore developmental theory when planning the fifth semester courses. A decision of this nature is so fundamental that it would require the vote of total faculty. However, the junior level team is responsible for determining the amount of emphasis and therefore the time to be allotted to a particular concept and/or hazardous event, and the individual who teaches the content is free to select the specifics, including class objectives, learning experiences, and evaluation measures. It is at this level that individual faculty creativity is encouraged.

SOURCES OF DATA FOR FORMATIVE EVALUATION

In the summative evaluation design, students and graduates were the major source of data. In formative evaluation, student opinions were solicited frequently and deserve consideration. When a program is first developing, however, it makes sense to place greater weight on the views of the experts. Achievement scores are hard data that cannot be contested, but opinions are subjective and influenced by so many variables unrelated to fact or even to knowledge that they must be interpreted with care. It seems more valid to place greater weight on the judgment of faculty, which is based on experience in education and nursing and on knowledge of educational principles as well as nursing theory, rather than succumb to the opinions of the novice, which are grounded in feelings and personal experiences.

Faculty Perceptions

Faculty input was secured informally through large and small group meetings and formally through questionnaires. Faculty really did not know how the new plan would work. Ideas had to be tested carefully, then retained, revised, or discarded. A built-in mechanism for ongoing evaluation was the series of meetings—unit teams, level teams, specialty groups, total faculty, small committees, etc.—set up to create and implement the new curriculum. These discussions were invaluable and resulted in appropriate changes, but needed to be supplemented periodically by data that could be objectively analyzed.

Formal Evaluation of Curriculum
Implementation by Faculty

As the end of the turbulent first year of implementation of the clinical nursing courses approached, it became obvious that both students and faculty had survived the change, that students and faculty had learned, and that there were aspects of the program that needed to be revised or further developed. In order to obtain reliable data, a tool was constructed by the junior level coordinator and the curriculum project committee. It asked for expressions of satisfaction or dissatisfaction with such varying elements of the curriculum as the crisis theory framework, the strands, the family study, the use of laboratory, various teaching strategies, and evaluative tools.

This instrument was probably too lengthy, which may explain in part why only nine of 12 faculty members returned it. However, it served the identified purpose by pinpointing the weaknesses as well as the strengths of the first year of implementing the new nursing courses. The findings provided a take-off point for subsequent discussion and planning. A year later, the questionnaire was shortened somewhat and adapted for use by faculty teaching the new senior year for the first time. Collecting faculty opinions in this manner ensured that everyone had an opportunity to express a carefully considered opinion on each point that was raised. Also, it gave the protection of anonymity, which was important at that stage when faculty were still unsure of themselves and each other.

By January 1977, four classes of students had completed the general education and supportive courses in the revised curriculum, but there were no evaluative data except informal comments. The follow-up questionnaire asked graduates to rate certain courses, but the opinion of faculty was also needed. If nursing is indeed an applied science and utilizes principles and concepts from other fields, it follows that faculty who teach nursing should be able to judge the adequacy of students' knowledge in those fields. Therefore, a tool was developed to solicit faculty opinions regarding the extent to which each of the supportive courses had met their expectations, that is, provided background for the nursing component. The results of this survey were shared with faculty teaching the courses as well as with School of Nursing faculty. The data obtained by this open-ended question were too limited to have any great significance when changes in the general education component were being considered, but it provided a basis for dialogue among faculty both within the School of Nursing and with other departments that teach nursing students.

When the school began an extensive self-evaluation in preparation for a National League for Nursing accreditation visit, more specific information was needed to identify areas in need of revision or further study. A questionnaire was thus constructed to elicit more detailed data from faculty. The items related not only to general education and supportive courses, but to many aspects of the nursing courses as well. A similar questionnaire was administered to junior and senior students so that their views could be considered before embarking on curriculum changes.

Evaluation of Instructional Materials by Faculty

Planning a completely revised nursing component, characterized by a variety of teaching strategies, necessitated reviewing a large amount of teaching materials including textbooks and media—the evaluator had to develop tools for this purpose. The textbook evaluation questionnaire was based on a paper by Langford, Stephenson, and Stanley (1973) as well as input from faculty. Tools of this type are valuable in helping inexperienced faculty determine what to look for when reviewing materials. Also, they provide a means of collecting and filing for future use data about books, media, and other instructional aids. The tools developed for this purpose early in this project were not widely used, probably because faculty were bombarded with so many tasks that only those of highest priority were attended to. However, the faculty member in charge of media has developed an excellent list of available material that is updated and distributed annually.

Course Evaluation by Students

Some notion of the difficulty of obtaining valid evaluations from students can be gleaned from the number of different tools that were developed for this purpose over a seven-year period. It seems logical to assume that a satisfactory tool would be used again and again rather than discarded after a short trial.

During the year that the first new course in the revised curriculum was taught, a published instrument, Class Activities Questionnaire by Steele (1969), was the basis for course evaluation efforts. This tool assesses teacher intentions and perceptions as well as student perceptions. It deals with cognitive emphasis based on Bloom's taxonomy, classroom conditions, and strengths and weaknesses of the course. Items related to specific courses were added to the basic tool. This instrument was designed to help teachers revise a course, not to measure its total worth, by comparing teacher intent to reality as perceived by teachers and students.

When this tool was developed by the program evaluator, it was intended to be used with appropriate modifications by all faculty for each course. During the past seven years a variety of tools has been developed, ranging from two pages to ten, ranging from completely objective items to completely open-ended ones. All of them served a purpose at the time they were used.

Whatever tool is selected or developed, several points are worth considering. First, do not overevaluate. Students get weary of it and fill out forms so lackadaisically that they are useless. (This became obvious when some students evaluated media in a course that used none and praised the use of role playing in a unit that was straight lecture.) Second, evaluation of a specific unit or even individual classes conducted immediately after the termination of the experience will probably elicit more meaningful data than a global evaluation of an entire course. Third, select the aspects of the course or unit that really need evaluating at a given time rather than trying to evaluate everything. For example, if faculty have tried something new or have concerns about particular aspects, select items that deal specifically with those areas and delete others. This will shorten the instrument and should provide more useful data. Fourth, sample student opinion if the class is large, rather than have every student fill out every questionnaire. Students seem to be more cooperative and take the tools more seriously if they are not asked to evaluate too often.

This chapter has aimed to illustrate a process rather than provide tools or an evaluation design for others to emulate. Reporting the findings is not necessary to fulfull that purpose, but failure to do so will leave the reader wondering about the results. Therefore, the remainder of this chapter will highlight the most significant findings. Detailed discussion of all of the data is beyond the scope of this book. More details are available in unpublished reports on file in the University of Connecticut School of Nursing (Brown, 1979; Brown, 1981).

FINDINGS

SAT Scores

The average verbal score of five classes graduating from the traditional curriculum was significantly higher than the average score of the first three new curriculum classes. This finding is in keeping with the national trend in scholastic aptitude scores. There is no reason to believe that it significantly influenced the outcomes of the curriculum. (The first class in the new curriculum had a significantly higher verbal score, but that difference disappears when the scores for all three classes are averaged.)

State Board Test Pool Examinations

Having developed a curriculum in which nursing content was reconceptualized and reorganized into a pattern that differed markedly from the traditional medical model approach, some very real fears remained: would the graduates pass State Board examinations? Would an integrated conceptual approach to nursing content adequately prepare students to pass five clinical specialty examinations developed from a very different perspective? No matter how effective a program has been in developing the many characteristics desirable in a professional practitioner, there remains the unalterable fact that licensure is mandated by law and is contingent upon passing the State Board Test Pool examinations.

It would be delightful to be able to report that graduates of the new curriculum scored significantly higher on State Board examinations than did their predecessors. Unfortunately, this was not the case. Except for the first class, which had a failure rate of only 2.73 percent, the difference between old and new curriculum classes was not significant. The fact that new curriculum graduates performed as well as their predecessors on the State Board examinations was encouraging to faculty, since other schools with newly-implemented integrated curricula had reported an increase in the failure rate. On the July 1979 examinations, the University of Connecticut pass rate was 92.6 percent, which exceeded the national norm of 84 percent for accredited baccalaureate programs.

National League for Nursing
Achievement Tests

Analysis of scores on National League for Nursing tests shows that new curriculum classes scored significantly higher on the medical-surgical application questions and on the sick child subtest. On the other hand, the traditional curriculum classes scored higher on psychiatric nursing and community health nursing. Analysis of the subtests revealed that scores in community health were lowered by the poor performance on the epidemiology and legal aspects sections. The implications of these findings are being considered as faculty discuss the strengths and weaknesses of the new program. On the National League for Nursing tests, as well as the State Board examinations, the University of Connecticut scores exceeded national norms in all areas.

Student Perceptions, Values, and Personality Traits

Many analyses have been performed on the data in this category but none of them have detected differences that can be attributed to curriculum changes. This finding is characteristic of educational research. One notable finding relates to the California Psychological Inventory. For all classes studied, the profiles were strikingly similar and well within one standard deviation of the female norms (the few male subjects in the study were excluded from the analysis because of the susceptibility of the CPI to sex differences). However, there is a difference between freshmen, sophomores, and seniors in all classes. For the most part, the senior profile is highest and the freshmen is lowest. Since the overall elevation of a profile indicates the level of effectiveness of a person's social and intellectual functioning, these data seem to merely confirm a process of maturation during the college years.

One of the purposes of administering the various tools was to identify characteristics predictive of success in nursing. Data from the Survey of Interpersonal Values were studied by Hayes as part of a doctoral dissertation. She concluded that further study was needed to demonstrate a relationship between personal characteristics and achievement. However, she did develop a prediction equation based on academic factors (Hayes, 1981).

Analysis of data from the Nursing School Environmental Inventory reveals one difference: seniors in the new curriculum scored significantly higher on intrinsic motivation. In other words, they felt that the school's environment did not pressure them into achieving or conforming. Instead, students were treated as adults and individual pursuit of knowledge was encouraged.

The above analysis focused on comparing the two programs. The next step will be to reexamine the data and determine how the new curriculum seniors view the school. For example, do they think the environment fosters independence? does it stimulate students to achieve? It may also be possible to use these data to identify items that seem to be useful and to develop new ones. In this way a tool can be constructed to collect the type of information that faculty think is important.

Follow-up Questionnaires

A large amount of data about graduates from the new curriculum was amassed using the follow-up tool. Undoubtedly, some of the findings will be analyzed further and reported by faculty in future publications. Some of these data will also be used in the future as a starting point for additional studies by graduate students and faculty. Just a few points will be made here.

First, the overall tone of the respondents is positive. The majority of the items on the performance evaluation section were rated good to excellent by the graduates and their employers, with the remaining items rated fair to good. Ninety-nine percent of the graduates rated their personal standards of care higher than (49%) or the same as (50%) that of other graduate nurses with the same amount of experience. Employer ratings are essentially the same. The strengths identified by both graduates and employers are: listening to patients and families; being accountable for his/her own practice; and explaining procedures and treatments to patients. Employers also gave high ratings to observing signs, symptoms, and changes in patients' conditions. The identified weaknesses are leading team conferences, initiating appropriate activity to change rules and regulations when necessary, and directing and evaluating the work of other nursing personnel (Brown, 1981).

Just as gratifying as these objective ratings are the many un-solicited comments that faculty hear when they are in clinical agencies with students and at professional meetings in various parts of the state. The comments indicate that people who have contact with University of Connecticut students are favorably impressed. More-over, employers are actively recruiting the graduates. There has been noticeable positive change in agency attitudes towards the University of Connecticut School of Nursing now that the new graduates are having an impact in various parts of the state; favorable reports are also coming from out of state.

None of this means that faculty are complacent. They will study the responses to many individual items on the follow-up tool to determine implications for curriculum change. For example, some of the ratings indicate that graduates feel less prepared in the care of the sick child than the adult. Also, some dissatisfaction with the general education requirements was noted. Each year a content analysis has been performed on the answers to the open-ended question at the end of the tool. These provide interesting insights that may influence future curriculum study.

An addendum to the follow-up tool questioned graduates of the new curriculum (classes of 1977 and 1978) about their use of crisis theory. Seventy-six percent reported that they were still using crisis theory as a conceptual framework for practice. The comments in response to questions about the use of the crisis theory framework are interesting, but too limited in number and content to be considered a valid evaluation of crisis theory as a model for practice. A systematic evaluation of the model is presented in Chapter 12.

SUMMARY

The evaluation plan initiated at the beginning of the project has served its purpose, in spite of problems and frustrations. Evaluative data gathered formally and informally from faculty, students, graduates, employers, and potential employers indicate that the curriculum design is sound. An integrated undergraduate curriculum based on a crisis theory model does work. Subsequent chapters describe the usefulness of the model for graduate education, practice, and research.

10

Articulation between Graduate and Undergraduate Programs

Janice A. Thibodeau

UTILITY OF A CONCEPTUAL MODEL

As Dorothy Reilly (1975) so emphatically points out, a school should have only one conceptual model or framework, regardless of how many programs it offers. The differences between programs lie in the levels of behavior specific for each program and the parameters of each program. As the model for the University of Connecticut School of Nursing, the crisis model guides the structure and development of both undergraduate and graduate program curricula and provides a means for articulation between the programs.

The three major model types in nursing are developmental, interaction, and systems. The crisis model is a developmental model focusing specifically on the developmental processes in the life of an individual and, therefore, utilizes life-span physiological, cognitive, and psychosocial theories for the basic theoretical formulation.

The purpose of this chapter is to give examples of how the developmental crisis model guides the articulation between programs rather than to provide a detailed description of the graduate program.

DIRECTION, SEQUENCE, PROGRESSION

Chin (1980) states that the concepts of direction, staging or sequencing, progression, and goals or potential are inherent in any developmental model. Each of these concepts is described below.

Direction

The process of development implies growth or change. Direction may be defined as a goal or endpoint or the degree of progress toward that goal. Hence, the model provides guidance for the development of the levels and terminal objectives of the program. Chapters 3, 4, and 6 illustrate this in relation to the undergraduate program. This chapter will show how the graduate program builds upon the base provided by the undergraduate program.

Sequence and Stage

A stage may be defined as a period of time on a developmental continuum that is qualitatively different from the stage preceding or following it. Graduate education is not merely more of what is provided in undergraduate education, but represents a qualitative difference. The concept of sequence provides a guideline for the general selection and placement of courses. The sequencing of courses described in Chapters 4 and 6 illustrates this point in relationship to the undergraduate program. This chapter shows how the undergraduate program influences the sequence of courses in the graduate program.

Progression

Progression refers to the progress from one stage to another or from one set of levels objectives to another. Chin (1980) refers to differentiation as a form of progression. Differentiation implies a generalist to specialist developmental progression as in the progress from undergraduate to graduate education. The graduate program builds upon the nurse generalist base of the undergraduate program to prepare specialists to function as nurse practitioners, managers, clinicians, and educators.

ARTICULATION BETWEEN UNDERGRADUATE AND GRADUATE PROGRAMS

Chater (1975) proposes a three-component structure for describing the elements of a conceptual framework: the student, the setting, an the subject. Chapter 3 discusses these in relation to the undergraduate program. Each of these three components will be examined as the basis for delineating the similarities and differences between the graduate and undergraduate curricula.

The Student

The typical learner in the undergraduate program is a late adolescent who entered college immediately following high school. Although there are nontraditional learners in this population, they form the minority rather than the majority of the student body. The learning theories and role of the faculty discussed in earlier chapters were formulated with the needs of this specific population in mind.

Since the goal of all education is the emergence of a self-motivated, independent learner, students are given increasing independence throughout the educational programs in accordance with their level of maturity and ability. Although undergraduate students have the opportunity for elective courses and input into the selection of learning experiences and the grading process, there is a definite developmental progression from undergraduate to graduate education.

Graduate students have the opportunity to select their areas of functional role preparation as well as their specialty areas. They have a higher percentage of elective courses than undergraduate students with fewer or less rigid course and credit requirements. The graduate student designs his/her own learning experiences based upon individual objectives and previous professional nursing experiences. This is in contrast to the individualization within prescribed clinical experiences that characterizes the undergraduate program. Also, many graduate level courses are graded by a student self-evaluation process as opposed to evaluation by a teacher.

The learner as an active participant, planner, and evaluator of her learning experiences is consistent with adult education learning theories, such as those of Knowles (1976), Havighurst (1972), and Hunt (1961). The typical learner in the graduate program is a young or middle-aged adult with a wide variety of experiences in nursing. This learner has a different set of developmental and career tasks than does the late adolescent. Thibodeau (1978) found that late adolescents are most concerned with the general knowledge necessary to secure a nursing position while the focus of the young and middle-aged adult is on specialized knowledge and skills that relate to specific career goals.

Perception of Event, Resources, Supports. Some specific examples related to components of the crisis model serve to further elucidate the differences between the characteristics and abilities of the undergraduate and graduate student. Since graduate education builds upon the foundations of undergraduate education, the graduate student possesses an increased understanding and ability to apply nursing theory, a broader and more in-depth knowledge of the behavioral and physical sciences than is true of the undergraduate student, and increased skill in the research process.

The undergraduate student's abilities in nursing research are typically concerned with questions relevant to nursing practice as delimited by his/her experiential base. The graduate student's concern with research transcends the field of clinical practice, generating research questions which have implications for nursing theory and the further development of nursing science. The research interests relate to nursing service and education as well as clinical practice.

The graduate student also develops a greater experiential base and the ability to test and evaluate a model of practice that is consistent with philosophical beliefs. The ability to synthesize nursing science with practical experience enables the graduate student to develop multiple insights into the intrinsic and extrinsic factors that lead to a client's perception of a hazardous event. Also, the graduate student has more skill and knowledge of resources to utilize in assessing and augmenting the client's resources and mobilizing situational supports systems.

Health Continuum. The wellness to illness to high-level wellness continuum is used by the crisis model to describe the health component. High-level wellness is a sophisticated and elusive concept to implement in practice and requires a sophisticated, competent learner as its executor. Dunn (1959) believes that in order to help others achieve a state of high-level wellness, helpers must know themselves very well and have resources of wisdom and maturity that are not in the usual repertoire of the adolescent learner.

The graduate program begins where the undergraduate program ends, at the more highly integrated level of wellness. Here the focus is on health maintenance, health promotion, and facilitation of high-level wellness. The undergraduate student typically focuses on one phase of the health continuum at a time. For example, when a client is ill, nursing care is directed primarily toward interventions related to the illness state although other phases are considered. The

UNDERGRADUATE STRANDS

GRADUATE COURSES

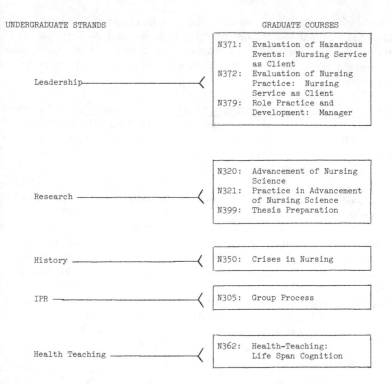

FIGURE 10-1. Relationship of strands to graduate courses.

graduate student may focus in depth on one phase of the health continuum but must keep a broad perspective in order to help the client achieve high-level wellness after recovery from illness. Interventions and planning by the graduate student are more inclusive, long-range and future-oriented than are those of the undergraduate student.

Crisis Continuum. The undergraduate student initially focuses on one phase of the crisis continuum at a time. For example, if the client is in a state of crisis, nursing interventions focus on that stage, although senior students begin to examine all phases of the continuum for selected clients. The scope of practice for the graduate student extends throughout the crisis continuum. In addition to management strategies aimed at the crisis stage, future planning for other clients in the pre-crisis stage are also considered. The undergraduate student cares for clients with selected developmental and/or situational hazardous events with somewhat predictable outcomes. The graduate student manages the care of clients with complex developmental and situational hazardous events with unpredictable outcomes.

Nursing Emphasis and Nursing Process. The undergraduate student typically focuses on man/environment interactions. For example, when caring for a client in crisis, the focus of nursing care is on the client and his family. The graduate student increases the focus of care to include implications for the health care system and the nursing profession itself. The interactions between man, environment, health, and nursing are considered in greater totality in graduate nursing education.

Because the assessment and planning phases have a broader perspective in graduate education, the implementation and evaluation phases are quantitatively and qualitatively different from undergraduate education. Graduate education emphasizes the evaluation phase of the nursing process. Nursing activities of graduate students include case finding, nursing diagnosis, and the planning of strategies for improvement of health care delivery. In addition, they design original assessment and evaluation tools, research studies, and guidelines for nursing audits, all of which are generated by a model of practice.

The Setting

Chater (1975) defines setting as the entire gamut of social, economic, political, and cultural parameters within the university and community at large. Since both programs are housed on the same campus, both have access to the same social, economic, political, and cultural advantages, and both feel the impact of existing constraints. Perhaps the major differences in the setting are the types of facilities and the geographic area utilized for clinical experiences. At the undergraduate level, experiences are provided along the entire wellness to illness to wellness continuum, and a variety of settings are utilized within a circumscribed distance from the main campus.

Since the focus of the graduate program is on high-level wellness, the majority of settings utilized are primary care settings. Also, the graduate program prepares students in a functional role (clinician, practitioner, teacher, manager) as well as in a clinical specialty (as opposed to the generalist preparation of the undergraduate student). Therefore, at the graduate level, the scope of agencies utilized is broadened to include experiences in the functional areas.

The geographic area utilized for graduate student clinical activities is much greater than that of the undergraduate program. The entire state of Connecticut and surrounding states are utilized as opposed to the 30 mile radius from campus utilized by the undergraduate program. The diversity of student objectives and selection of experiences to meet individualized learning needs necessitates an expansion of the territory employed.

The Subject

A brief description of how subject matter is ordered by the crisis model might demonstrate how the model provides the framework for articulation between the undergraduate and graduate programs. Undergraduate education is generalist in function and, for all students, contains theory and clinical experiences related to all phases of the health-illness continuum. Graduate education is specialist in nature and experiences need not focus on the entire continuum but on providing more depth at any given point.

Since the focus on the graduate level is on high-level wellness rather than the entire health-illness continuum, the course content and clinical experiences are geared to assessment and enhancement of wellness rather than illness intervention. A student may also elect to concentrate experiences in one of the crisis phases—pre-crisis, or post-crisis—rather than in all three.

Organization of Content

The simple to complex continuum serves as the guideline for organization of content. Beginning at the undergraduate level, theory and practice focus first on developmental hazardous events, then situational hazardous events, and lastly on combined developmental/situational hazardous events with somewhat predictable outcomes. In the graduate program, all advanced theory courses and clinical practicums focus on combined, complex developmental/situational hazardous events with nonpredictable outcomes.

Core Courses. Core courses are required of all students in the graduate program and give the foundation needed in the advanced areas. The core courses for the curriculum are "Conceptual Models of Nursing Science," "Crisis in Nursing," and "Nursing Research."

While the undergraduate program is based upon the crisis model, the students do not undertake an analysis of the crisis model per se. In the course, "Conceptual Models of Nursing Science," which graduate students take in the first semester, the crisis model is specifically analyzed as a model for nursing practice. This model is compared and contrasted with other nursing models. Life-span developmental theories, which form the underpinnings of the crisis model, are also analyzed in greater depth than in the undergraduate program. After analysis and evaluation of several nursing models, the graduate student can decide which model he/she will select for implementation in his/her own practice.

In the course, "Crises in Nursing," trends and issues relevant to the health care system and to the nursing profession are examined in greater scope and depth than in the undergraduate program. Students must carefully analyze how crises in the nursing profession affect their own practice of nursing and design strategies to deal effectively with actual and potential crises.

In the two nursing research courses, the crisis model is analyzed from the perspective of how a conceptual model generates research questions and guides the nursing research process. As in the models course, the research implications of the crisis model are compared and contrasted with other nursing models. In the first research course, taken in the second semester, the focus is on the research process and design of a research proposal. In the second level research course, taken in the third semester, students implement their research proposals and report their findings either through a formal thesis or a written report accompanied by an oral presentation. The undergraduate research strand focuses on preparing the student to become an intelligent consumer of research; this focus is expanded in graduate education.

Specialty Areas. The crisis model also mandates organization of the traditional clinical specialty areas in a way different from the medical model. Since the crisis model is a developmental model, an age-span approach is a logical outcome. Specialty areas are divided along the age-continuum with emphasis in some cases on a particular type of crisis and/or type of recipient of nursing care. The specialties are:

Childbearing/Childrearing Families
Adults in Bio-physical Crisis
Persons in Psychosocial Crisis
The Older Adult
Families Acorss the Life Span
The Community as a Client
Nursing Service as a Client

Functional Areas. Students may elect to become prepared as teachers, practitioners, clinicians, or managers. In all courses related to these options, the implications of the crisis model are studied with regard to practice, education, and research. For example, students who elect to prepare as teachers analyze the curriculum of the University of Connecticut School of Nursing as an example of how a conceptual model guides curriculum development. Students are then expected to design a unique curriculum using the crisis model or another nursing model of their choice. The crisis model is used as the basis for contrast and comparison of all other models. In the role course related to teacher preparation, students can actually implement their models.

Strands. In the undergraduate curriculum, strands are content areas related to nursing concepts that are common to all courses and, therefore, present in varying degrees throughout the entire upper division major. In the graduate program curriculum, each of the strands has been expanded into one or more separate, advanced graduate level courses (see figure 10-1). The leadership strand has been expanded to a series of courses designed to prepare nurse managers.

SUMMARY

A conceptual model, such as the crisis model, provides concrete guidelines for curriculum development and evaluation as well as for articulation between a school's graduate and undergraduate programs. The crisis model is a developmental model which provides guidelines for the direction, sequence, and progression of the curriculum. The concepts of student, setting, and subject provide the basis for delineating the similarities and differences between graduate and undergraduate curricula. The crisis model is an exciting model to use because of its future orientation and emphasis on growth, high-level wellness, and the maximum potential inherent in each individual. This model poses a satisfying challenge to practitioners, educators, and researchers who attempt to apply it in their practice.

11

Using Conceptual Frameworks in Nursing Practice and Research

Jacqueline Fawcett
Evelyn Hayes

This chapter focuses on the use of conceptual frameworks in nursing practice settings and as guides for nursing research. Emphasis is placed on specific applications of the crisis theory conceptual framework.

CONCEPTUAL FRAMEWORKS AND
NURSING PRACTICE

Although the abstract nature of a conceptual framework places it several steps away from nursing practice, conceptual frameworks clearly influence practice. As explained in Chapter 2, each conceptual framework reflects a world view that presents a particular orientation or perspective of reality and therefore provides certain guidelines for clinicians' activities.

It is probable that most nurses have implicit private images of nursing practice, that is, their own frames of reference that influence their assessment of clients' behavior, their nursing diagnoses, and their choice of intervention strategies. Conceptual frameworks are now making these private views explicit and are identifying commonalities among various nurses' ways of looking at people and their environments, wellness and illness, and application of the nursing process (Reilly, 1975). Conceptual frameworks can thus help the clinician identify the focus of nursing, structure knowledge relevant to nursing, and set boundaries for nursing practice.

Moreover, these frameworks offer a consistent view of phenomena in the everchanging world of practice (Hagemeier & Hunt, 1979).

Despite the advantages, many nurses and student nurses find it difficult to use a conceptual framework until they become accustomed to its vocabulary and special slant on nursing. Certainly, the abstract nature of conceptual framework concepts can result in vague boundaries among concepts as well as among the categories of any one concept. Moreover, abstract concepts are not always clearly defined. These facts may be responsible for some of the difficulty nurses experience when trying to use a conceptual framework. This is indeed the case with many baccalaureate students when they first become acquainted with nursing.

New graduates may also experience some difficulty using a conceptual framework. Hagemeier and Hunt (1979) found that although 84 percent of the 69 baccalaureate graduates responding to their survey questionnaire indicated they could articulate a conceptual framework, only 66 percent said they were using one to guide their practice. These authors speculated that "this discrepancy could be attributed to other factors in the new graduates' work environment" (Hagemeier & Hunt, 1979, p. 547), such as their lack of confidence in their technical skills and other practitioner behaviors. In a one year follow-up study of University of Connecticut graduates (classes of 1977 and 1978), 71 percent indicated they were using the crisis theory framework in their practice. Those who were not using it included as the reasons poor staffing, not enough time, and task-oriented jobs.

Difficulties with the use of a conceptual framework are also encountered by nurses who have been practicing for some time. This is probably because they have been using their own images of nursing or because they have been practicing with a medical model as their primary frame of reference.

Even those faculty who participate in the development of new conceptual frameworks for curricula often experience difficulty when first using these formalized views of nursing. To paraphrase White and Coburn (1977, p. 646), the transition from a traditional, and implicit, conceptual framework with which one feels comfortable and competent to one that represents an explicit and completely different approach to nursing can provoke a great deal of anxiety. Fortunately, this situation usually does not last for long. As Broncatello (1980) commented, "Much like the development of any habitual behavior, [using a conceptual framework] initially requires thought, discipline, and the gradual evolvement of a mind set of what is important to

observe within the guidelines of the model. As is true of most habits, however, it makes decision making less complicated" (p. 23).
Some of the difficulties encountered by the faculty of the University
of Connecticut School of Nursing when they began to implement the
crisis theory conceptual framework within an integrated curriculum
are described in previous chapters. Other problems as well as successes are discussed in articles by White and Coburn (1977) and
Murdock (1978).

While the difficulties engendered by use of a new conceptual
framework are real and must be acknowledged, the advantages of its
use are far more outstanding. As noted in Chapter 2, conceptual
frameworks of nursing provide a distinct focus for nursing and can
increase nurses' confidence that what they are doing is nursing.
Furthermore, since conceptual frameworks consider the whole person in interaction with the environment, nursing's goal of dealing
with clients in a holistic manner is facilitated. A hypothetical example of the use of the crisis theory conceptual framework in a practice situation will help to illustrate this point.

A Practice Example

Jane and David Johnson's first contact with the Visiting Nurse Association occurred when they attended the annual health fair and had
their blood pressures taken. At 39, Jane's readings were within
normal limits, but David (42) had a markedly elevated reading of 180/
100. Prior to this time, David and Jane had been unaware of his
elevated blood pressure or the implications of this condition. Because of the abnormal reading they became part of the Visiting Nurse
Association caseload.

The crisis theory conceptual framework provides guidelines
for nursing interventions in each stage of the crisis cycle. In the
pre-crisis stage, nursing interventions focus on augmenting resources for the purpose of averting a crisis, or at least decreasing
the impact of the event on the client. As part of the assessment of
David, the nurse discussed his perception of the hazardous event—
elevated blood pressure—and identified risk factors that were operating in this situation. These included family history of cardiac
disease; a stressful, sedentary job; erratic dietary habits; and
smoking. David also indicated that when he was stressed, he worked
harder and smoked more cigarettes. It also became evident that, in
addition to many risk factors, David had a reservoir of resources—

motivation to achieve goals; a supportive wife, family and friends; an unremarkable health history to date; steady employment; above-average intelligence; and financial solvency.

On the basis of this initial assessment data, the client and nurse mutually formulated a plan with goals that included such areas as realistic perception of high blood pressure, anticipatory guidance, health teaching, resource management, utilization of previous coping behaviors, and/or development of new coping behaviors. For example, through health teaching David and Jane gained a more realistic perception of the situation as well as the risk factors that contributed to it. Together they identified supports that could be mobilized to decrease the number and/or intensity of the risk factors. Specifically, Jane would prepare nutritious meals based on sample recipies, and both would determine and carry out an exercise program. While aware of the hazards of smoking, they were not motivated to work on this factor at this time. Both agreed to work on reducing these selected risk factors for the next month and then to evaluate their efforts.

In this instance, interventions of anticipatory guidance, increased supports, and health teaching did not avert a crisis for the Johnsons. Within a short time, David experienced a myocardial infarction and was hospitalized. The reader will recall from Chapter 3 that the concept of crisis relates to the client's reaction to the event, rather than the event itself. In the case of David's myocardial infarction, there was a biological crisis due to loss of patency of coronary blood vessels—the hazardous event. In addition, David perceived the event as a crisis in his life.

According to the crisis theory model, if the client experiences a crisis, total nursing support may be indicated. However, the nurse must be alert to the changing needs of the client, allowing and encouraging him to assume increasing responsibility in decision making and in actual care as his condition warrants it.

Emotional support of the client is indicated in any stage of the crisis model. During the crisis phase, many interventions are also directed to life maintaining activities. In David's case, interventions were associated with loss of patency, of regulation, sensory motor loss, and loss of relationships. As losses contributing to a crisis are stabilized, the client takes an increasingly active role in decision making. This could begin with realistic choices about the timing of personal care activities and the selection of food preferences and progress to the resumption of responsibility for future planning.

As David began his biological recovery from the myocardial infarction, he and Jane began to participate in a cardiac rehabilitation program designed to prevent future biological insults as well as to help develop the coping mechanisms necessary for resolution of the psychosocial elements of the crisis. At this point, the nurse needs to be alert to the client's capabilities and resources and to foster independence and interdependence.

Upon discharge from the hospital, David returned to the active caseload of the Visiting Nurse Association. Based on the crisis theory conceptual framework, nursing interventions during post-crisis focus on supporting the client through to a healthy resolution whereby he returns to a level of wellness at least equal to his pre-crisis state. More specifically, the goal is that the client will grow as a result of the crisis and will, therefore, reach a higher level of wellness. In David's case, nursing interventions focused on his growth potential, with health teaching receiving the major emphasis. Principle areas for health teaching are compliance with prescribed regimens, developing appropriate coping mechanisms to deal with stress, and change in life style.

Through experiencing the crisis of a myocardial infarction, David Johnson did attain a level of wellness that was higher than before his illness. Jane and David now have a broader health knowledge base as well as insight into the importance and integration of preventive health behaviors. In addition, their diet and activity levels are now more appropriate. David has made decisions and taken actions to reduce the stress in his work situation and set some realistic goals regarding his life's ambitions.

The preceding example illustrates how the crisis theory conceptual framework directs the nurse's attention to many aspects of the client situation. The various components of the framework guide observation of not only presenting symptoms of disease but also of other factors that contribute to the total client situation. Regardless of the stage of crisis, the nurse must make accurate assessments and nursing diagnoses, and intervene in a manner that capitalizes on all the client's resources.

CONCEPTUAL FRAMEWORKS AND
NURSING RESEARCH

Conceptual frameworks alone will not provide the specification and the verification of knowledge needed to make nursing a scientific enterprise. Only research and the concomitant development of theory can do that. While the abstract nature of a conceptual framework places it a few steps away from nursing research, the framework clearly influences all aspects of scientific research. The world view provided by the framework orients the researcher to certain phenomena and to certain ways of conducting research. As discussed in Chapter 2, study variables are derived from the abstract concepts of the framework: the basic assumptions of the framework lead to more specific statements of relations among study variables and then to testable hypotheses. Conceptual frameworks thus have the "basic purpose of focusing, ruling some things in as relevant, and ruling others out due to their lesser importance" (Williams, 1979, p. 96). In an indirect manner, then, conceptual frameworks are tested by research; the findings of this research can be used by clinicians in the practice setting.

The Relation of Research and Theory to Practice

Conceptual frameworks influence research. In much the same way, they influence theory development. Chapter 2 included a discussion of the distinctions between conceptual frameworks and theory and advanced the position that nursing theory is best derived from conceptual frameworks of nursing. Also noted in that chapter was the fact that theory is required for specific actions of clinicians in particular clinical situations. This theory can be developed only through research. Indeed, the sole purpose of scientific research is "to understand and explain natural phenomena" (Kerlinger, 1979, p. 280), that is, to build and test theory. No matter how goal-directed a study may appear to be, no matter how atheoretical it may look, its only real purpose is to generate, refine, expand, or refute theory. Thus, research influences practice through its generation of theory.

It may be recalled from Chapter 2 that theories describe, explain, or predict relations among phenomena and that, in practice disciplines, theories may also prescribe the actions of clinicians. The generation, refinement, and expansion of these different types of theory is accomplished by different types of research. One way to distinguish types of research is in the application of the basic-applied dichotomy.

Basic research builds or tests theory by studying relations among variables. It is done with little or no thought about use of results in practical situations and is therefore not conducted to achieve any practical goal. Basic research may yield descriptive, explanatory, or predictive theory. Such research derived from the crisis theory conceptual framework could, for example, focus on verification of clinicians' observations that the state of acute crisis is usually limited to six weeks (Caplan, 1964). Research could begin by describing the amount of time required to resolve a crisis given different developmental and/or situational hazardous events. Next, variables thought to explain the time limits could be investigated. Finally, predictions of the time required for crisis resolution given certain circumstances and certain hazardous events could be established.

In contrast to basic research, applied research is directed toward solution of specific practical problems in particular situations or settings. This type of research is done with the expectation that a problem will be solved, a condition ameliorated, or a process improved. Clearly its aim is to achieve an explicit goal (Kerlinger, 1979). Applied research is most likely to generate what Dickoff and James (1968) called prescriptive or situation-producing theory, that is, theory that specifies goals, prescriptions for action, and the parameters or scope of the theory in terms of client conditions and clinical settings. Prescriptive theory presupposes theory at the lower levels however. This means that applied research is appropriate only after descriptive, explanatory, and predictive theories have been developed through basic research.

The development and testing of nursing care strategies that prevent crisis following the birth of a child is one example of applied research derived from the crisis theory conceptual framework. Before such studies can be undertaken, however, much basic research needs to be done to build the theoretical structure. Theory describing the crisis of parenthood is needed, as is theory explaining the influence of various factors, such as family supports and community resources on development of this type of crisis. Predictive theory dealing with the effect of nursing interventions on people's coping mechanisms is also needed.

In nursing, the basic-applied dichotomy is often translated as the theoretical-clinical dichotomy. This can be a misleading distinction however. When attached to a study, the adjective "clinical" means only that research takes place in a clinical setting, not that it is an investigation of nursing practice. In fact, as Downs (1979) noted, either basic or applied research may be conducted in a clinical setting. The emphasis on clinical research in nursing seems to stem from clinicians' needs for theory to direct their actions. However, any leap to nursing practice research from an unsound base of lower level theory will accomplish nothing. Indeed, practice based on no theory or on an unvalidated theoretical structure is just as much trial and error guesswork as that based on no research at all. It is thus imperative that descriptive, explanatory, and predictive theories are validated before research aimed at building and testing prescriptive theory begins. This is because scientific practice requires a firm foundation of reasons for clients' responses to situations and events. And these reasons are discovered only by repeated studies that test alternate explanations and that finally establish the most accurate theory.

For those who think most current nursing research has nothing to do with nursing practice, a careful review of the nursing literature should reveal that even the most basic theoretical nursing studies arise from and ultimately relate to nursing practice problems. If it were different, the research could not be considered nursing research. The key word is time—it takes a great deal of time for knowledge to be sufficiently developed and validated for practice. Indeed, the establishment of a body of knowledge directly related to practice is a very slow process, requiring the tenacity and persistence of researchers who may work for years on minute pieces of giant puzzles. Consider that it took perhaps 100 or more scientists over 100 years to identify and describe DNA, and that only now, more than 25 years after the discovery of its structure, are explanations regarding its role in human life forthcoming.

The slow and cumulative nature of scientific research and the generation of knowledge needed for practice is seen in the following discussion of the basic/applied research continuum. This differentiation of types of research was described by Gage (1963) as a paradigm for educational research and was later adapted for nursing by Kramer (Chater, Kramer, & Tone, 1975) and Downs (1979). The first category on the continuum is basic scientific research—content indifferent. Here, research is highly abstract and is aimed at building or testing theory that will describe, explain, or predict phenomena. This type of research generally considers the relation between variables; the setting for the study and the type of study subjects are usually not especially relevant. Any number of situations could be used to test the relation being investigated. Indeed, subjects may not even be humans.

Examples of this type of research derived from the crisis theory conceptual framework would be studies seeking to validate the relational statements presented on pp. 56–57 of Chapter 3. One such study might investigate the relation between coping behaviors and problem solving by examining subjects' behavior when asked to solve a complex puzzle. The nature of the problem and the particular coping behaviors would not be of special interest. In fact, several studies should be conducted to establish the variety of situations in which the relation is demonstrated. Some studies might even use laboratory animals to examine this relation in terms of such physiological coping behaviors as adrenal hypertrophy.

The next category is basic scientific research—content relevant. This type of research includes studies that attempt to define the knowledge needed for practice, but does not necessarily arise from a specific need in the practice arena, as in the case of applied research. Such studies continue to test and refine theory developed in the first category, and clarify relations among variables in situations more closely related to practice, such as a simulated clinical unit. Often, however, research methods and controls would be unrealistic in the actual clinical setting. Research derived from the crisis theory conceptual framework that fall into this category include studies of how people cope with different hazardous events. For example, one of a series of studies related to the crisis of parenthood might be directed at descriptions of people's responses to a videotape recording of a crying baby. From a different viewpoint, this type of research could also focus on the nurse. For example, a study might be directed toward descriptions of the nurse's reactions to clients experiencing a loss of patency as manifested by severe chest pain.

The third category is investigation of practically-oriented nursing problems. This step on the continuum deals with nursing research problems that are at least conceptually similar to those found in clinical settings. The research may take place in a simulated clinical area or in an actual one. Subjects may be healthy volunteers or actual clients. Here, research based on the crisis theory conceptual framework could use volunteer subjects to explore, for example, adrenal hormone levels or cardiac and respiratory rates after exposure to a simulated situational hazardous event. Or volunteer subjects in a computerized laboratory setting could be given instructions about how to calm a crying baby and then could be tested for their ability to stop the crying of a doll programmed to respond to appropriate actions. The focus here is clearly on nursing practice problems and the theory needed for understanding phenomena related to such problems. Unless this type of research is built upon theory developed by basic scientific research, however, findings will reveal only pragmatic relations among variables. While especially attractive to the clinician seeking solutions to pressing clinical problems, such relationships do not rest on a firm foundation of validated theory and therefore are of little scientific value.

Another research category is clinical experimentation. This involves experimentation on nursing practice problems in controlled situations. Here the emphasis is placed on testing the effects of different nursing interventions on client outcomes. Often the experiments take place in specially prepared settings, such as clinical demonstration units. Real patients are generally used as subjects. An example of this research category within the crisis theory conceptual framework is McGillicuddy's (1977) study of differences in the behavior of children in rooming-in and non-rooming-in hospital situations. Study findings indicated that the children in rooming-in settings exhibited more mature behavior posthospitalization than did the children in the non-rooming-in settings. McGillicuddy concluded these findings lend support to the crisis theory proposition that "given support and/or intervention during a time of crisis one can, in fact, make positive changes in behavior" (p. 74). Another example in this category would be testing certain structural supports and resources necessary to create the environment conducive to caring for the terminally ill at home.

At this point on the continuum, research based on theory that has been developed and refined in the preceding steps can begin to progress to the development of nursing practice strategies. Such new ideas, approaches, and methods are further tested and refined in the next research category, clinical trials. Here, knowledge leading to development of practice innovations is transferred from the simulated or demonstration units to a representative set of clinical agencies. The researcher then has to prepare nurses in these settings to use the new strategies to solve actual problems. Data for this type of research include the nurses' abilities and willingness to apply the innovation appropriately as well as clients' response. Any deviations from the expected outcomes for clinicians or clients are examined to determine if the new strategy needs to be refined or if further study at one of the preceding steps on the continuum is needed. Research in this category might focus on the clients' and staff's responses to instituting rooming-in for all hospitalized children. Or a study might determine in-patient and out-patient health agency personnel's responses to a home care program for the terminally ill client.

The final category of the basic/applied continuum is the wide dissemination of research findings. At this point, demonstrations, workshops, and seminars as well as use of the professional and lay news media help to promote acceptance and uniform application of practice innovations. The most appropriate and effective use of this category is dissemination of new strategies that have been systematically investigated in the preceding research categories. Unfortunately, as Downs (1979) noted, this is not always the case: "The extent to which . . . practice innovations have actually been subjected to the scientific rigor of the preceding steps is often more questionable than the ordinary professional consumer realizes" (p. 85).

An example of this situation is the current interest in prepared childbirth. From the perspective of the crisis theory conceptual framework, prepared childbirth classes are a form of anticipatory guidance for labor and delivery. Although this method of childbirth has been enthusiastically embraced by many health professionals and a large majority of pregnant women and their partners, little research supports its superiority over other methods. In fact, studies by Goodwin (1970), Hott (1972), and Windwer (1977) have found no significant differences between prepared and unprepared childbearing couples on such measures as self-concept, locus of control, and social desirability.

Research needs to be directed toward identifying and describing the specific benefits of this widely accepted practice. This is especially important in light of recent study findings that suggest parents have adverse reactions when their plans for a prepared childbirth experience are not realized (Fawcett, 1981; Marut & Mercer, 1979). This example serves to illustrate an outcome of adopting a practice modality that has not been based on a firm foundation of theory building and theory testing research. It seems crucial, then, that clinicians question the validity and consequences of new practices before they adopt them.

Perhaps the most meaningful way to distinguish types of research is on the basis of the amount of knowledge about a topic already available and validated. This is especially so if the knowledge is directly derived from the conceptual framework of interest. Then connections among conceptual framework, theory, research, and practice begin to fall into place. Payton's (1979) categories of research are helpful here and fit well with Dickoff and James' (1968) hierarchy of theory.

Descriptive research, which attempts to identify and describe the specific characteristics of particular people, groups, situations, or events, is required when nothing or very little is known about the particular phenomenon in question. This type of research generates descriptive or factor-isolating theory. Correlational studies are appropriate when the essential characteristics of study variables have already been adequately described. The aim of this type of research is to explain relations among variables. Thus, it generates explanatory or factor-relating theory. Predictive research is needed when relations among concepts are adequately explained and causal relations are of interest. Predictive or situation-relating theory is generated by this type of research.

Payton does not have a research category that corresponds to prescriptive or situation-producing theory. He notes that descriptive, correlational, or predictive research frequently provides the knowledge needed for practice. Furthermore, Beckstrand (1978) claims that nursing does not need specific prescriptive theory in the sense advocated by Dickoff and James (1968). Rather, she takes the position that descriptive, correlational, and predictive research generates all the scientific knowledge needed for nursing practice, and that the ethical knowledge of nursing provides the prescriptions needed for action in clinical situations.

An example of Payton's categories is seen in a series of studies identified by a group of staff interested in parental response on first seeing their child following cardiac surgery. Initially, research at the descriptive level would be necessary to identify behaviors exhibited by parents. This research would be followed at the correlational level with the identification of those factors that influenced this parental response. The next level of research, predictive, would aim to identify those factors that were important for prediction of the parental response. Identification of significant nursing interventions and development of a general nursing care plan is the desired outcome of the fourth level of research, situation-producing.

Another example is found with community health nurses' concerns about client compliance with prescribed regimens. Research at the descriptive level would include identifying behaviors of compliant and noncompliant clients. Factors that influenced these behaviors would be identified at the correlational level of research. Next, situation-relating research serves to identify factors considered important in the prediction of these behaviors. At the situation-producing level, development of appropriate nursing intervention and general nursing care plan are the goals.

It should be obvious by now that research derived from the crisis theory conceptual framework is needed in many areas. Four areas of possible research that clearly require systematic investigation are risk factors, crisis behaviors, client role, and the growth-promoting potential of a crisis. Identification of risk factors has been discussed in previous chapters. Initially, descriptive research is needed to identify risk factors for various hazardous events.

Also of interest is the relation between the number and type of risk factors and the severity of the impact of the hazardous event. Crisis behaviors must first be described. Subsequent concerns to be addressed include the relation of perceived crisis and receptivity by the client to interventions. A related area is the relation of perceived crisis and the ability to seek intervention. Antecedent to this is the perception of the event since a given event may be a crisis for one individual and not for another. Questions of research interest are: must certain critical factors be present for an event to be perceived as a crisis? If so, what are these essential components?

The client role is another aspect of the crisis theory conceptual framework. Behaviors descriptive of the role of client need to be identified. Later studies might focus on the effects of the client role on recovery rates. Related areas include the degree of nursing satisfaction derived from working with clients (rather than patients) and the acceptability of the client role to the consumer, nurse, family, and others.

Growth, the most unique concept of the crisis model, has much potential for research. What are growth behaviors? What factors influence these behaviors and are predictive of them? What determines transference of coping behaviors to future events?

It was pointed out earlier that conceptual frameworks help the researcher to select relevant variables and guide the formulation of theoretical statements and testable hypotheses. Although the crisis theory conceptual framework has generated numerous theoretical statements, many of which were presented in Chapter 3, few of these statements have been tested in a systematic manner. Given the paucity of validated knowledge, an appropriate research strategy is description of framework concepts. The following examples of research using the crisis theory conceptual framework illustrate the application of descriptive research strategies to the developmental hazardous event of parenthood and provide data that could be used to formulate descriptive theory.

Research Examples

Parenthood has repeatedly been characterized as a developmental hazardous event that can precipitate a crisis (Benedek, 1959; Robischon, 1967). Numerous empirical studies present contradictory findings regarding the number of couples who experience a crisis following the birth of their child as well as the magnitude of any crisis that does occur (Dyer, 1963; Hobbs, 1965; Hobbs & Cole, 1976; Hobbs & Wimbish, 1977; LeMasters, 1957; Russell, 1974). This area, then, seemed appropriate for additional descriptive research using the crisis theory conceptual framework.

Fawcett's (1977, 1978b) longitudinal study of couples' body image changes during and after pregnancy provided an opportunity to explore the extent of the crisis of parenthood as well as the length of time until resolution of any crisis that occurred. One year after the birth of their child, 74 couples who participated in the body image study were asked to complete a questionnaire regarding the crisis of parenthood. Sixty-eight of the wives and 67 of the husbands in the sample completed the questionnaire, which is presented in figure 11-

Thirty wives indicated they had not experienced a crisis following the birth of their last child. Twelve of these women were

The birth of a child is sometimes considered a crisis, that is, a time of upset and disorganization, for a family. Do you think you experienced a crisis following the birth of your last child?

_____Yes _____No

If you answered Yes, at what time following the baby's birth did things seem to return to a more usual state for your family?

_____ 2 weeks after the baby's birth

_____ 4 weeks after the baby's birth

_____ 6 weeks after the baby's birth

_____ At another time (please explain)

What factor(s) do you think contributed to the crisis?

Please describe, as best you can, how you felt during the time of crisis.

If you answered No, what factors do you think helped you to avoid a crisis?

FIGURE 11-1. Crisis of parenthood questionnaire.

primiparas, 13 had their second child, four their third child, and one her fourth. Thirty-eight wives indicated they had experienced a crisis after the birth of their last child. Of these, 25 were primiparas, nine had their second child, two their third, and two their fourth. Forty-eight of the husbands indicated they had not experienced a crisis, while 19 indicated that they had. Twenty-three of the first-time fathers said they had not experienced a crisis, while 13 of these husbands had experienced one. Chi-square analysis of the data revealed no statistically significant relation between parity and experience of crisis for either wives or husbands. Additional chi-square analyses revealed no significant relation between social position or years of marriage and the experience of crisis for either spouse.

The data revealed also that of the 38 wives who experienced a crisis, 16 indicated that family life returned to a more usual state within six weeks after the baby's birth. However, nine wives said it took up to six months for resolution of the crisis, and the remaining 13 wives experienced crisis for up to one year postpartum. Of the 19 husbands who had experienced a crisis, eight said the crisis was resolved within six weeks, five said it took up to six months, and the remaining six husbands said the crisis continued for up to one year after the baby was born.

Tung (1977) performed a content analysis of these couples' responses to the questions dealing with factors contributing to the crisis of parenthood and feelings during the time of that crisis. Many of the wives reported feeling fatigued, depressed, angry, and emotionally labile during the time of crisis. They also felt inadequate, disillusioned, anxious, and disorganized. Husbands reported many of the same feelings although to a lesser degree. Both wives and husbands reported feeling overwhelmed. Wives attributed this feeling to increased household chores while husbands cited increased financial burdens. Two wives and one husband indicated that they felt jealous of their spouse after the baby's birth. Interestingly, one wife and four husbands reported feeling optimistic throughout the period of crisis.

An additional content analysis was performed on the couples' responses to the question dealing with factors that helped them to avoid a crisis. Most wives and husbands cited external support from family members, friends, and hired help as major factors. They also noted the positive influence of planned pregnancies and preparation for the new baby. This was especially so for the multiparous couples, who commented that they knew what to expect after having had one or more other children. Many couples also attributed the lack of a crisis to the strong positive relationship they had with each other. This finding is interesting because Tung (1977) found no evidence of a relation between occurrence of a crisis and marital adjustment [determined by Spanier's (1976) Dyadic Adjustment Scale] for either wives or husbands.

These data suggest that crisis is experienced more frequently by women than by men after the birth of a child. Apparently, demographic variables such as social class, years of marriage, and parity have no influence on the occurrence of the crisis of parenthood, nor does the marital relationship. The feelings reported by those who experienced a crisis are similar to the general characteristics of a crisis previously described (Caplan, 1964) as well as to reported responses to the crisis of parenthood (Hobbs & Wimbish, 1977). However, since many couples indicated the crisis of parenthood extended well beyond the six-week limit usually associated with a crisis, it may be that this particular crisis requires more time for resolution than do crises precipitated by other hazardous events. This area clearly requires additional research. Furthermore, the data presented here regarding factors that helped to prevent a crisis following childbirth suggest that anticipatory guidance and general support would be effective nursing interventions during pregnancy and postpartum.

D'Amato's (1978) study of postpartum nursing intervention is another example of research within the crisis theory framework. She investigated the effect of scheduled home visits and telephone contacts during the first six weeks postpartum on the occurrence of crisis in a sample of four couples. The Crisis of Parenthood Questionnaire was used to describe crisis events. In addition, Hobbs' (1965) checklist was used to determine the extent of crisis.

Three of the couples in the sample indicated they did not think they had experienced a crisis following the baby's birth, while the other couple said they had experienced one. However, according to the scoring protocol for Hobbs' checklist, three couples were placed in the "slight crisis" category, while one couple was in the "moderate crisis" category. There thus seems to be a discrepancy between the one item measure of crisis and a more extensive questionnaire on various behaviors common to a crisis response to parenthood. Results of D'Amato's content analysis of the questions dealing with factors contributing to the crisis, and crisis behavior for the one couple indicating they experienced a crisis, are similar to Tung's (1977) findings. Similarly, D'Amato's findings for the question dealing with factors that helped avoid a crisis correspond to those reported above.

The sample size and design of this study prevented any conclusions regarding the effect of nursing interventions on the occurrence of the crisis of parenthood. D'Amato did find that one couple who had experienced a crisis required additional contacts during the postpartal period. This couple reported that the crisis was resolved by the sixth postpartal week. All couples in the study indicated that the scheduled contacts, as well as the knowledge that they could contact the investigator if necessary, were helpful and beneficial.

The preceding examples of research using the crisis theory conceptual framework suggest that a great deal more research is required to more fully test the propositions of the crisis formulation cited in Chapters 3 and 12. Little research has been done thus far. The framework has been adopted uncritically by many health professionals, and practice has been based on intuition more than on the results of empirical research. The danger here is that the use of this conceptual framework as a guide for practice could become as ritualized and unscientific as practice guided by trial and error. An extensive program of nursing research would help to prevent such an undesirable situation from developing.

INTEGRATING RESEARCH AND PRACTICE

D'Amato's (1978) study is a good example of how research and practice within a given conceptual framework can be combined. Her nursing interventions could easily be adopted by nurses caring for families during the childbearing period. Since the research instruments take little time to complete, data could be easily collected from families in the course of a home visit. Analysis of the data would provide the information needed to describe the efficacy and effectiveness of selected types of anticipatory guidance and general support during the postpartum period.

Given the paucity of crisis theory research, it is worth noting that most nursing care activities conducted within this conceptual framework could be linked to other research in much the same way that D'Amato's work is linked to other studies. The systematic description of outcomes would provide the needed data for theory building within the context of this conceptual framework.

SUMMARY

Although conceptual frameworks are needed to provide a uniquely nursing perspective to nursing practice, and research is needed to move nursing practice away from automatic, ritualized procedures and toward thoughtful, systematic processes, neither a conceptual framework nor any study will ever be able to tell clinicians exactly what to do. Rather, conceptual frameworks and research together influence ways of thinking about and interpreting phenomena. This is because conceptual frameworks are too abstract and too general to direct specific actions in particular situations and because the probabilistic nature of scientific research itself generates "knowledge under conditions of uncertainty" (Selltiz, Wrightsman, & Cook, 1976, pp. 47-48). Furthermore, in nursing not just empirical knowledge but also esthetic knowledge (the art of nursing), ethical knowledge, and knowledge of the therapeutic use of self are needed to help the clinician decide what to do in a given situation (Carper, 1978). Carper's own words clarify this best: "Nursing . . . depends on the scientific knowledge of human behavior in health and in illness, the esthetic perception of significant human experiences, a personal understanding of the unique individuality of the self and the capacity to make choices within concrete situations involving particular moral judgments" (p. 22).

12

Evaluation of the Crisis Theory Conceptual Framework

Jacqueline Fawcett
Eileen Murphy

This chapter will present an evaluation of the crisis theory conceptual framework. The evaluation will be organized according to the criteria for evaluation of conceptual frameworks discussed in Chapter 2. These criteria are stated in the following questions.

1. Are the biases and values underlying the conceptual framework explicit?
2. Does the conceptual framework provide complete descriptions of all four essential concepts of nursing? Do the basic assumptions completely link the four concepts?
3. Is the internal structure of the conceptual framework logically consistent? Does the conceptual framework reflect the characteristics of its category type? Do the components of the conceptual framework reflect logical translation of diverse perspectives?
4. Is the conceptual framework socially congruent? Does it lead to nursing activities that meet social expectations or do the expectations created by the framework require societal changes?
5. Is the conceptual framework socially significant? Does it lead to nursing actions that make important differences in the client's health status?
6. Is the conceptual framework socially useful? Is it comprehensive enough to provide general guides for practice, research, education, and administration?

7. Does the conceptual framework generate empirically testable theories? Do tests of derived theories yield evidence
   in support of the framework?
8. What is the overall contribution of this conceptual framework
   to the body of nursing knowledge?

EXPLICATION OF BIASES AND VALUES

The biases and values of the crisis theory conceptual framework
have been made explicit by the faculty of the University of Connecticut School of Nursing. The framework clearly reflects the faculty's
value of a wellness perspective, as can be seen in the emphasis on
intervention during the stage of pre-crisis. The faculty also values
a holistic approach to the person, which is demonstrated by a focus
on the person as an integrated biological, psychological, social, and
cultural being.

The emphasis placed on growth in the crisis theory conceptual
framework indicates the faculty's bias toward viewing crisis as a
positive event in a person's life, rather than a negative one. This
bias toward growth is translated into nursing actions that assist the
client to identify his or her own needs and the resources available to
meet those needs, thus facilitating client independence rather than
dependence. The client is viewed as an active participant in health
care, not simply as a reactor to events occurring in the environment.

Essential Concepts and Linking Statements

Given the abstract nature of conceptual frameworks, the descriptions
of the person, the environment, health, and nursing goals and process set forth in the crisis theory conceptual framework appear to be
adequate. However, as noted in Chapter 3, the extension of the idea
of growth in crisis theory to the biophysical component of person in
the conceptual framework is not fully explained.

The statements linking person, environment, health, and nursing do not leave any gaps among these concepts. In fact, as can be
seen in Chapter 3 (pp. 56–57), the four essential concepts of nursing
are linked in each of the three stages of crisis (pre-crisis, crisis,
post-crisis) outlined in the conceptual framework.

Logical Consistency

The crisis theory conceptual framework is logically consistent. This can be seen in the diagram of the relationships among the concepts of the framework presented in figure 12-1. This diagram follows Hardy's (1974, 1978) method of assessing the internal logical consistency of a formulation. Hardy indicated that this is most easily done by assigning symbols to represent concepts and by diagramming the relationships among the concept symbols. The resultant diagram facilitates detection of logical errors.

Figure 12-1 depicts the relationships of the various concepts of the crisis theory conceptual framework. The symbols for these concepts are identified in the verbal linking statements listed below.

1. Persons exist in a state of dynamic equilibrium with their environments.

    $P \longrightarrow E$

2. Nursing actions are taken to strengthen this interaction.

    $N \xrightarrow{+} P \longrightarrow E$

3. Hazardous events cause a disruption in this dynamic equilibrium.

    $HE \longrightarrow DDE$

4. This disruption in dynamic equilibrium evokes problem-solving behaviors.

    $DDE \longrightarrow PSB$

5. Adequate problem-solving behaviors lead to problem solution.

    $APB \longrightarrow PS$

6. Nursing actions augment problem-solving behaviors.

    $N \xrightarrow{+} APB \longrightarrow PS$

7. Problem solution leads to a new dynamic equilibrium at the same level of functioning.

    $PS \longrightarrow NDE$

8. Inadequate problem-solving behaviors lead to crisis.

    $IPB \longrightarrow C$

9. A state of crisis calls forth additional resources.

    C ——→AR

10. Appropriate additional resources lead to crisis resolution and the learning of new problem-solving behaviors.

    AAR ——→CR & NPSB

11. Nursing interventions help to mobilize and utilize appropriate additional resources.

    N —$^+$—→AAR ——→CR & NPSB

12. New problem-solving behaviors result in a new dynamic equilibrium at a higher level of wellness.

    NPSB ——→HLW

13. Ineffective additional resources lead to increased tension.

    IAR ——→IT

14. Increased tension may lead to maladaptation.

    IT ——→M

15. Maladaptation may lead to a new steady state at a lower level of wellness.

    M ——→LLW

16. Nursing actions assist in the achievement of the highest level of wellness possible.

    M ——→LLW + N ——→HLW

17. Increased tension and/or maladaptation may lead to major disorganization.

    IT & M ——→MD

18. Nursing actions reduce the effects of major disorganization when recovery is impossible.

    N —$^-$—→MD

Classification of the Conceptual Framework

It may be recalled from Chapter 2 that conceptual frameworks of nursing are classified as developmental, interaction, or systems

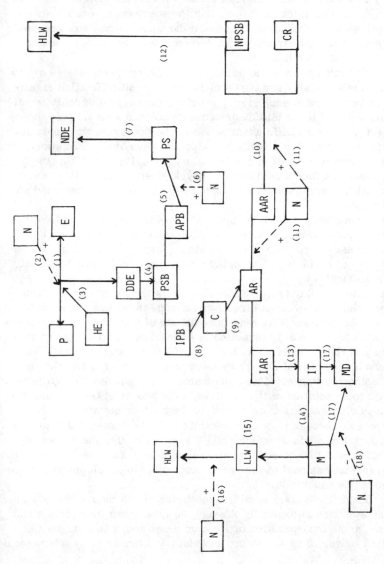

FIGURE 12-1. Diagrammatic representation of the crisis theory framework.

217

orientations to knowledge. The crisis theory conceptual framework may be classified as developmental. Chin (1980) states that developmental orientations "center around growth and directional change . . . they assume that there are noticeable differences between the states of a system at different times, that the succession of these states implies the system is heading somewhere, and that there are orderly processes that explain how the system gets from its present state to wherever it is going" (p. 30).

The conception of the person passing through the stages of pre-crisis, crisis, and post-crisis, with the identification of possible resolution at each stage, provides the general developmental orientation of the crisis theory conceptual framework. (See figure 3-1.) A more specific examination of the developmental orientation of the framework is provided by a comparison of the framework with the characteristics of this orientation, as outlined by Chin (1980). He identifies the major terms of developmental orientations as: direction, identifiable state, form of progression, forces, and potentiality.

Chin (1980, pp. 30-31) notes that developmental models postulate directional change in the person. He outlines the direction of change as: (a) some goal or end state (developed, mature), (b) the process of becoming (developing, maturing), or (c) the degree of achievement toward some goal or end state (increased development, increase in maturity) (p. 31). The crisis theory conceptual framework clearly addresses directional change in postulating growth or continued disorganization as the outcome of a crisis. Furthermore, as seen in figure 3-1, direction is maintained in all stages from pre-crisis through crisis to post-crisis. The curriculum content elaborates on directional change by incorporating Erikson's (1963) developmental stages. Thus, the framework identifies the goal or end state to be solution of the problem in the pre-crisis stage, and continued disorganization or growth in the post-crisis stage. The process of becoming is also considered in the conceptual framework through Erikson's developmental stages. Finally, the degree of achievement toward some goal or end state is addressed through the nursing assessment of the person according to developmental stages and crisis resolution.

Identifiable state is addressed in the crisis theory conceptual framework most explicitly through the idea of stages of crisis and through the incorporation of Erikson's developmental stages, as noted above. Both the stages of crisis and Erikson's developmental stages fit Chin's (1980, p. 31) criterion for this developmental model characteristic by being qualitatively different from one another.

Chin (1980, pp. 31-32) explains that four forms of progression through developmental change are possible. First, unidirectional development may be postulated, such that "once a stage is worked through, the client system shows continued progression and normally never turns back" (p. 31). Second, developmental change may take the form of a spiral, so that while return to a previous problem may occur, the problem is dealt with at a higher level. Third, development may be seen as "phases which occur and recur . . . where no chronological priority is assigned to each state; there are cycles" (p. 32). And fourth, development may take the form of "a branching out into differentiated forms and processes, each part increasing in its specialization and at the same time acquiring its own autonomy and significance" (p. 32). The crisis theory conceptual framework assumes a spiral form of progression more than any other. This is seen in the idea that if a crisis is successfully resolved (that is, if growth occurs), the person has added to his or her repertoire of problem-solving mechanisms and will be more likely to successfully resolve future crises.

Chin (1980, p. 32) defines forces as "causal factors producing development and growth." The crisis theory conceptual framework addresses forces when it identifies the hazardous events that have the potential to upset the individual's steady state. Developmental or situational hazardous events are thus seen as the forces which require the person to change and grow if crisis resolution is successful. Moreover, the crisis theory conceptual framework views nursing interventions as forces, in that interventions help the person toward crisis resolution and, therefore, toward growth.

Potentiality, the overt or latent capabilities of the person for developmental change (Chin, 1980, p. 32), is clearly addressed in the crisis theory conceptual framework through the major concept that the person has the innate capacity to grow toward a maximal level of wellness. Moreover, the framework identifies the person's problem-solving mechanisms as the means by which the capability for growth is realized.

LOGICAL TRANSLATION

The crisis theory conceptual framework reflects an organismic world view of the relation between person and environment (Reese &

Overton, 1970). This view denotes a model of the person as an active organism in continuous interaction with the environment. The person is seen as influenced by and influencing events in the environment, not as just a passive respondent to environmental stimuli. The organismic view is characterized by the concept of holism, such that the person is an integrated whole, more than a simple sum of parts. This perspective is demonstrated in the conceptual framework by the idea that the person is active in developing problem-solving mechanisms and actively seeks help from health professionals during times of crisis. Moreover, curriculum content focusing on Erikson's (1963) developmental stages attests to the emphasis on the organismic view. The holistic concept is addressed in the conceptual framework in the description of the person as an integrated biophysical-psychosocial-cultural being.

The faculty of the University of Connecticut School of Nursing has attempted to keep the organismic view consistent throughout the curriculum. While their attempts are largely successful, some mechanistic views are represented, especially in the use of Selye's (1950) ideas of stress and in use of stimulus-response theories of learning motor skills (see Chapter 3, pp. 50–51 and Chapter 7, pp. 111-112). The mechanistic view, which is logically incompatible with the organismic perspective, denotes a model of the person as a passive, reactive organism responding to external environmental stimuli. In this view, change is seen as the sole result of external forces (Reese & Overton, 1970). Thus, the conceptual framework requires logical translation of the contrasting organismic and mechanistic views wherever they occur in the curriculum while some concepts must be redefined so that all reflect the same basic world view.

Social Congruence

Exemplified by Florence Nightengale's edict—"nurse the sick, not the sickness" (Dolan, 1978)—the focus of nursing has traditionally rested upon the individual and not on his illness. This emphasis on the person rather than on the problem per se is one of the strongest aspects of the crisis theory conceptual framework. The originators of crisis theory repeatedly emphasize that it is the reaction of an individual to a problem that determines the development of a crisis, not the problem itself. Thus, any approach to providing nursing care within this framework must focus upon the individual—his perceptions, strengths, needs, and resources—rather than merely focusing upon the pathogenetic features of the problem.

The provision of client-centered as opposed to problem-centered nursing care would appear to facilitate the individualization and personalization of the care delivered to each client. The impersonal, uncaring, and routinized services offered to many clients have long been deplored by the public. Since the crisis theory conceptual framework directs nurses' attention to the unique perceptions and responses of each person facing an overwhelming problem, nurses' attempts to help him to attain and maintain health will have to be tailored to his particular needs and resources.

The consumers of health care services have frequently expressed their dissatisfaction with being treated as passive recipients rather than as active participants in their own care. Because the crisis theory conceptual framework emphasizes that interventions are geared toward the augmentation of clients' problem-solving abilities, their active participation in the process is expected. In other words, interventions are not meant to solve problems for clients, but rather with them. In addition, because successful intervention is accompanied by the acquisition of new problem-solving behaviors, ability for self-care in the future is enhanced. Thus, it may be concluded that the crisis theory conceptual framework is congruent with present social expectations of nursing care.

Social Significance

From its inception, the crisis theory conceptual framework emphasized the goal of intervention as prevention rather than merely amelioration or maintenance. Activities guided by the goal of prevention would insure that nursing actions would significantly enhance the quality of life, not merely reduce disease. Based upon the assumption that successful crisis resolution results in growth, this approach directs nurses to interventions that have an impact on the individual's future level of health and not just on an episode of immediate concern. Because the framework deals with all life events, both developmental and situational, nursing intervention becomes a significant force within the total life experience, not just a measure reserved for disease.

Caplan (1964) noted that the kind of help that a person gets during trouble is a vital determinant of the outcome of his crisis. This framework places emphasis upon the importance of adequate, appropriate intervention and also suggests the unfortunate results of failing to provide such interventions. The significance of intervention in determining outcomes is strongly emphasized by this framework.

Although empirical observations of outcomes using crisis theory support the assertion that the use of this framework does make significant positive differences in the client's health status, there is virtually no scientific research to be offered as evidence. Such research is vitally needed.

Social Utility

The crisis theory conceptual framework has demonstrable utility for nursing practice, education, administration, and research.

The broad perspective of clinical nursing practice provided by the framework is especially noted in the framework-directed attention to all life events related to health. Thus, nursing efforts encompass the entire health-illness continuum, rather than being limited to episodes of illness. Moreover, while the framework does not directly predict the development of a crisis in a given individual, it does call attention to those events that have the potential for influencing health. Therefore, the framework is useful to nurses in all clinical practice setting, regardless of specialty orientation.

In addition to this broad perspective, the conceptual framework provides direction and organization at the care-giving level. Parameters of client assessment and intervention are clearly delineated, as outlined in figure 3-1 and as explained in Chapter 3. The utility of the conceptual framework for practice is also discussed in Chapter 11.

The utility of the crisis theory conceptual framework for education is demonstrated in the many chapters in this book devoted to curriculum. The curriculum grid clearly outlines the areas for curriculum content derived from the conceptual framework. Moreover, as explained in Chapter 10, the framework has demonstrated usefulness in directing the articulation between the undergraduate and graduate programs of the University of Connecticut School of Nursing.

The crisis theory conceptual framework has also begun to demonstrate its usefulness in administrative nursing activities. The Graduate Program of the University of Connecticut School of Nursing includes several courses which incorporate nursing management activities within the context of the conceptual framework.

The utility of the conceptual framework for guiding nursing research is clearly described in Chapter 11. As noted in that chapter, the basic concepts of the conceptual framework provide areas for descriptive, correlational, and experimental nursing research.

Generation of Theory

A few efforts at deriving a legitimate theory from the crisis theory conceptual framework have been made (Bloom, 1963; Halpern, 1973, 1975). Since these efforts have not been particularly successful, the framework remains a set of abstract concepts and general linking statements. However, the many relational statements of the framework may certainly be considered the precursors of theories, once concepts have been more clearly explicated and operationally defined.

Contribution of the Framework
to Nursing Knowledge

Clearly, the crisis theory conceptual framework has been useful in guiding the development of a well-organized nursing curriculum. The concepts of the framework have provided an organizational schema for nursing content that delineates a logical sequence of courses, guides selection of relevant course content, provides a consistent way of looking at client situations, and outlines types of nursing interventions appropriate for assisting clients in attaining a maximal level of wellness.

A special contribution of this framework is the idea that crisis is not a negative aspect of life, but rather can be growth-promoting. Moreover, the framework guides nurses to consider both well and ill persons as legitimate clients in need of nursing care. Finally, the framework directs the nurse to look at the person's existing coping mechanisms and to help the client develop new mechanisms as needed in a given situation.

13

Curriculum Model Applied to Student Practice: Nursing Management of the Adolescent Hemophiliac

Pamela Stacey

Editor's Note. This chapter was adapted from a paper written when the author was a seventh semester student. The focus of the chapter is the development of a holistic nursing protocol for the adolescent hemophiliac. In the eighth semester, the author utilized the protocol in the nursing management of a hemophiliac client. This chapter is included here to demonstrate a student's utilization of the curriculum model as a guide for her practice. In addition, it provides a more detailed illustration of the application of the crisis theory model to a client situation than do the illustrations in previous chapters.

In order to fully comprehend the application of crisis theory to the hemophiliac adolescent, it is necessary to understand the illness as well as the characteristics of adolescence. To most people, the mention of hemophilia conjures up images of ancient royal families in which this sex-linked genetic disease was passed on from generation to generation. They picture pathetic creatures who must live sedate, isolated lives in order to avoid possible injury and life-threatening bleeds. In actuality, however, hemophiliacs in today's society may look just like you and me, and, with the advent of factor replacement therapy, they may also have a very similar life style.

  Hemophilia is not one entity in itself; instead it is a group of congenital, hereditary conditions affecting the coagulative properties of the blood (Weiss, 1970). The disease is transmitted as a sex-linked trait on the X-chromosome. Therefore, aside from rare cases of spontaneous mutations or carrier female/hemophiliac male combinations, which create a hemophiliac female, all hemophiliacs are male. In each form of this disease an essential clotting factor of the blood is either absent or deficient (Strauss, 1972). The most common form of hemophilia, and the one discussed in this chapter, is factor VIII deficiency, or Hemophilia Type A. In this form of hemophilia, blood clotting is prolonged or nonexistent due to a gap in the intrinsic pathway of blood coagulation at the level of factor VIII. In these individuals the frequency and severity of bleeding is in direct proportion to the percentage of functionally available factor VIII in their blood (Aledort, 1971). The relation of factor VIII levels to overt symptomatology in the three classes of Hemophilia Type A (Aledort, 1978) is as follows:

> Mild hemophilia (5-50% factor level): (1) Bleeding only after severe insult; (2) Coagulation screening tests normal or low normal.
> Moderate hemophilia (2-5% factor level): (1) Infrequent spontaneous hemorrhages; (2) Significant hemorrhages after minor trauma; (3) Prolonged PTT; (4) Rarely pass coagulation screening tests.
> Severe hemophilia (less than 1% factor level): (1) Frequent spontaneous hemorrhages all their lives; (2) Coagulation screening tests always abnormal.

Examining these percentages, it is easy to see that the effect of hemophilia on an individual's life style is not only related to the type of hemophilia, but also to its degree of severity. The hemophiliac must always face the reality of possible bleeding crises. However, with the development of purified factor VIII concentrates, cryoprecipitates, and fresh frozen plasma, prophylactic therapy or rapid infusion of these solutions greatly decreases the risks of bleeding (van Eys, 1977). In the past, the only treatment for bleeding episodes consisted of whole blood transfusions which often led to fluid overload and death. Now, however, with these concentrated products of factor VIII, large amounts of the factor can be quickly infused and the bleeding can be confined. This greatly decreases such complications of hemophilia as hemarthrosis, paresis, and paralysis of motor and sensory nerves (Dressler, 1980).

As a result of this improved technology, hemophiliacs are now being taught home therapy. They learn to detect the signs and symptoms of bleeding and infuse themselves with the appropriate product.

This allows hemophiliacs to have greater independence in their care, a more mobile life style, and a feeling of control over their disease and their individual destinies (van Eys, 1977).

The benefits of home therapy are of particular importance to the adolescent. It is in the adolescent years that the identity is formed and there is thus a critical need for independence and self-direction at that time (Tiedt, 1972). The adolescent period is a time of breaking away from the family and developing a sense of self. It is in this time span, from roughly age thirteen to nineteen, that individuals must decide who they are and where they are going. Parental influence begins to have a diminishing effect and the peer group and idols increase in significance. Body image and physical appearance reach a peak of importance, and mature interest in the opposite sex is aroused. All the events which occur in the adolescent years feed into the permanent identity structure of the individual and subsequently shade the remainder of his life. It is these aforementioned areas that are the most vulnerable to irreversible damage in the adolescent years when illness or disease complicate development. As hemophilia and the adolescent are discussed, therefore, these areas will be specifically addressed.

PRE-CRISIS

Hemophilia: A Hazardous Event for the Adolescent

Hemophilia can be viewed as a hazardous event in all three realms of the individual—physical, social, and psychological. Physically, hemophilia is a significant hazardous event because it can cause exsanguination, hemarthroses, and other major complications. These physical hazards pose a significant risk for the adolescent because the teenage years are a time of increasing activity. Team sports become an important part of the teenager's life: for the teenage hemophiliac, some of these sports must be forbidden. For example, football, which could cause painful ankle bleeds, may have to be replaced by a more gentle sport like badminton (Ross, 1979).

Parents, doctors, and nurses must aid the adolescent in restricting activities which may be dangerous for him, while still striving to maintain a normal life. Too much restriction and overprotection on the part of the parents might have the effect of causing rebellious and risk-taking behavior. Hence, the goal for the nurse working with these patients and families should be to assist them in achieving a realistic perception of the situation and a program of activities that is both safe and rewarding.

The manner in which hemophilia is a hazardous event in the social life of an adolescent is really quite obvious. Hemophilia, a chronic, treatable, but incurable condition, poses a significant threat to the life style of an adolescent. Like the adolescent dia-betic who cannot give up junk food because he might lose face with his peers, the adolescent hemophiliac also faces social sanctions. Being unable to take risks and occasionally requiring hospitalization may make the teenager feel isolated and may also cause him to fear his condition.

The best way to avoid or overcome these social problems is through educating the adolescent about his illness. "One way to pro-mote such adaptation is to provide the child with ever-increasing knowledge concerning his condition and those methods that he may use to assist in his own care" (National Hemophilia Foundation, 1972, p. 3). This is where the professional nurse can be of unlimited value. The nurse must not only teach, she should also assist the family members to understand the complexities of the condition.

Lastly, hemophilia represents a hazardous event psychologi-cally to the adolescent. As mentioned previously, adolescence is the time during which the identity is formed. The body image, a major portion of an individual's identity, is also in its formative stage. This represents a significant problem for the adolescent hemophiliac. This teenager is aware that he is not the same as his peers, nor will he ever be. He wonders what will happen to his body and how he will cope with these changes (Tiedt, 1972). Many of the alterations that occur in the body because of hemophilia will affect the adolescent's future plans and relationships. This is a heavy psychological burden to bear and thus creates many psychological hazardous events. The unique characteristic of hemophilia, however, that makes it even more psychologically devastating than other conditions, is summed up as follows: "It may be easier for an individual to adjust to a dis-ability which is constantly present like blindness or deafness than to hemophilia where the person is outwardly normal except during epi-sodes of bleeding" (The National Hemophilia Foundation, 1972, p. 1). Consequently, even if the adolescent is fortunate enough not to have any overt deformities of hemophilia, he is still not spared the psy-chological effects imposed by the disease. Hence, these patients need counseling and conscientious preventative care to ease adjust-ment and prevent crises.

Intrinsic and Extrinsic Factors
Predisposing the Adolescent Hemophiliac to Crisis

The first intrinsic factor to consider is that of the extent of factor VIII deficiency. The greater the deficiency of factor VIII (and, thus, the more severe the hemophilia), the greater the chance of a bleeding episode—a crisis. Therefore, the nurse working with the severe hemophiliac adolescent should be sure that the patient is aware of the symptoms of a bleed, so that crises may be quickly resolved (Aledort, 1978).

A second intrinsic factor, closely related to the first, is that of the site of the bleed. When the bleed does occur, its site is a major determinant of whether there will be a crisis or not. Bleeds into closed spaces such as the structures of the head and neck, perineum, and femoral triangle are more crisis-provoking than ones into the arm (Liggins, 1976). Adolescent hemophiliacs will probably tend to have more problems with this intrinsic factor since their activities often cause serious bleeding.

The third and last intrinsic factor to be considered is that of the adolescent's psychological ability to cope with and adapt to his condition. An adolescent does not yet have an adult's sophisticated coping patterns and this may cause him to enter into a crisis much faster. He is still trying to acquire such qualities as self-control, independence, ability to defer gratification, and acceptance of the self—attributes that can protect an individual against the impact of such a sudden and unexpected blow (Tiedt, 1972).

In smmary, it can be stated that there may be certain unique intrinsic factors which make adolescent hemophiliacs less able to ward off a crisis than other age groups. A major focus for assessment for the nurse working with adolescent hemophilacs should include the degree of factor deficiency, the usual site of bleeds, and the adolescent's coping abilities. Only through awareness of these intrinsic factors can the plan of care be truly specific to that client.

Extrinsic factors which predispose the patient to a crisis are generally easier to change than intrinsic ones. An example of an extrinsic factor that can and should be altered by the nurse working with the client is that of proximity to medical care. This may be a particular problem with the adolescent who does not drive or have access to public transportation. With the advent of home care and self-infusion therapy, this factor may not be a problem. For patients who do not want to manage their own therapy, however, it is necessary to have a readily accessible center where they can go in the event of a bleed. If the patient is vehemently opposed to home therapy and is far removed from hospitals, the nurse or other health professional should ensure that doctors or clinics are equipped to care for the hemophiliacs in their community. It is a proven fact that the longer the delay in treatment, even for minor bleeds, the more serious is the damage to joints, nerves, and vessels (Aledort, 1978). Thus, accessible treatment should be a priority in the plan of care.

A second extrinsic factor that must be discussed with the adolescent hemophiliac is that of employment. Activity levels and sports have already been mentioned as predisposing the adolescent hemophiliac to a crisis, but jobs can often be just as hazardous. Many adolescent boys find employment which requires lifting, climbing, and other sources of potential trauma to the body. This can lead to crisis-provoking bleeds into joints, which remain as permanent deformities. A further problem with employment is that many potential jobs are denied to hemophiliacs because of their condition (Aledort, 1975). This factor can be devastating to the adolescent both psychologically and financially. This is a time when the adolescent obtains his first job and if serious difficulties arise in this developmental task, future vocational goals may be irreversibly damaged. The professional nurse must therefore work to educate the public about the capabilities of the hemophiliac and try to dispel any ancient myths which still exist.

Lastly is the factor of finances. Hemophilia is a costly condition in terms of its chronicity, exacerbations, and the difficulty of finding employment. Although some public funding is now available to aid this population, monetary concerns still represent a significant problem because therapy is extremely costly (Dietrich, 1977). This problem rarely affects the adolescent directly, since the family pays the bills, but it does influence the type of care that he can receive. The nurse should refer the families to sources of funding. She might also participate in action to increase federal and state funding to aid patients and families afflicted with this disease.

Coping Mechanisms Used by Patient and Family

The next area of concern for the nurse is that of the coping mechanisms employed by the patient and his family. The nurse must assess whether these coping mechanisms are effective or if they are hinderin treatment. It is then her responsibility to either support the client in his pattern of coping or to assist him in attaining a more realistic view of his condition.

The most common coping mechanism utilized by the recently diagnosed adolescent hemophiliac is that of denial. This is not unique to hemophilia—denial is often utilized as an initial defense mechanism when an illness is discovered. Some adolescents use denial because they resent the intrusion the condition makes in their lives. This denial may be manifested by refusal to recognize symptoms or to change their life styles. Sometimes patients, particularly adolescents, will deny the need for treatment because they are embarrassed or fearful of a hospital or clinic visit (Weiss, 1977). They may be more willing to accept treatment if the alternative of home therapy is offered.

Denial is also a coping mechanism frequently used by the family of the hemophiliac adolescent. Parents may deal with distressing facts or emotions by pretending that they do not exist and by wanting to know as little as possible about hemophilia. When this coping mechanism is no longer sufficient, as, for example, when a bleed occurs that cannot be denied, parents may turn to anger, guilt, or martyrdom. It has been found that one of the best ways to help the family adjust to this condition is through group sessions (National Hemophilia Foundation, 1972). The nurse should help the family to locate these groups through the National Hemophilia Foundation or assist them in forming their own groups in their community. Before such groups are available, she should personally help them to explore their feelings.

Another coping mechanism used by both adolescents and children who are ill is regression. Unlike the adult, who primarily uses denial during illness, the adolescent often couples regression with denial to protect himself from the reality of his illness. This reaction is not necessarily negative as long as it does not impede the treatment of the disease or the adolescent's normal growth and development. The nurse should be supportive of the adolescent while trying to assist him in accepting his condition. She should try to maintain a continuous and stable relationship in which the patient is given acceptance and the opportunity to discharge his energies in a manner that fosters self-control. She should accept this behavior, allowing for regression, but with the expectation of growth (Tiedt, 1972). For the adolescent, hemophilia does not have to retard growth and development but may actually be a learning experience.

Internal and External Resources

Lastly, in the pre-crisis stage, internal and external resources shall be explored. It is hard to actually list which resources each individual adolescent hemophiliac will utilize, but some common ones will be highlighted here. As stated earlier, the adolescent does not have the sophisticated, psychological defense mechanisms that the adult may possess. Although he can use regression and denial to a certain extent, additional internal and external resources are needed. One internal resource that the adolescent hemophiliac has is youth. In general, such complications of hemophilia as joint deformities, kidney disease, and factor antibodies do not become well-established until after adolescence (Boone & Spence, 1976). There is therefore still hope of warding off these potential crises by prompt detection and early treatment of bleeding episodes. To accomplish this goal, the nurse working with the adolescent and his family should make sure that they understand the signs and symptoms of bleeding episodes and the need for prompt treatment. This topic will be discussed more fully under patient teaching in pre-crisis.

An additional internal resource of the adolescent hemophilic stems from the nature of hemophilia itself. With the advent of improved preventative care, much of the adolescent hemophiliac's life can be relatively healthy. Occasional bleeding episodes are inevitable but, for the most part, the adolescent hemophiliac under medical care can enjoy a seemingly normal existence. "Unlike the child whose bleeding is associated with a concommitant disorder, the child with hemophilia is otherwise well" (Liggins, 1976). This factor can allow the adolescent to gradually assimilate his condition into his identity structure. He can adjust to his disease at his own pace because overt symptoms are concealed. This is a helpful internal resource for adolescents with whom acute illness usually signals psychological and social crises.

External resources available to the adolescent hemophiliac are abundant. Since the adolescent is most likely still residing with his parents, the family can be one of his greatest resources. " . . . [T]he psychic health of the child ill with hemophilia depends on complete and sincere family involvement" (Aledort, 1978). Thus, one of the first areas that the nurse should assess is the patient-family relationship. She should ensure that there is open, two-way communication and reinforce the family for its support.

Other available external resources are the medical team, nurses, counselors, factor concentrates, and the National Hemophilia

Foundation. Factor concentrates will be discussed later, in the crisis section. External resources which are common to many conditions will not be discussed here so that the focus can be on the National Hemophilia Foundation. This organization is an external resource of limitless value to the hemophiliac patient and his family. Its programs, their publications, and their lobbying for funds and programs have had a tremendous impact on the type of care available to hemophiliacs today (Aledort, 1978). All professional nurses should be aware of this precious resource for their hemophiliac clients so that they can benefit from this organization's services.

Nursing Intervention in Pre-Crisis

Now that the characteristics of the patient in the pre-crisis stage have been reviewed, nursing interventions and patient teaching in that stage will be presented. Patient teaching in pre-crisis is an immense topic due to the surge of recent knowledge about the condition and the growing realization of the importance of preventative care. A good place to begin is with patient education on the basic nature of the disease. It is a well-established fact that a critical factor in both the patient and the family's acceptance of hemophilia is knowledge of the condition (Bittner, 1974). The nurse should teach the family how the disease was transmitted, the pathophysiology, treatment, complications, and the importance of preventative care. She should dispel myths and evaluate the patient and family's understanding of the disease before she begins her teaching. An open, understanding atmosphere should be maintained between the family and the nurse so that questions and concerns can be freely expressed. It must be remembered that the hemophiliac is a member of the community. Therefore, teachers, nurses, and administrators should be included in the teaching plan. They should be taught that unusual care and undue restriction of activity are unnecessary (Liggins, 1976). The main goal to strive for should be as normal a life as possible for the hemophiliac adolescent.

The next topic for patient teaching is to describe bleeding episodes. The most important aspect to stress first is that most bleeding episodes are mild and that the child will not bleed to death from a minor cut. After the patient and family seem comfortable with this issue, the teaching can proceed to the signs and symptoms of a bleeding episode. The patient and family should learn that, although superficial bruises are seen easily, deep bleeding can occur in the muscles without outward, visible signs. They should know that the following symptoms indicate that the patient is probably hemorrhaging and should be treated immediately: movement of a limb is restricted; pain or numbness is present; a joint feels boggy, or hard and hot (Bittner, 1974). Reassure the family and the patient that prompt treatment usually prevents permanent deformity and that the blood will soon be reabsorbed by the body. As an additional precaution, all hemophiliacs should wear identification chains (National Hemophilia Foundation, 1974). Nurses should ascertain whether their hemophiliac clients wear these tags, and, if not, help them to obtain them.

The next area of patient teaching deals with one important aspect of preventative care—how to prevent hemorrhages. Hemorrhages from trauma are very difficult to prevent, but if a clear plan of allowable and forbidden activities is developed it may decrease this risk. Since it is important for the adolescent to participate in his own care, it would be beneficial to jointly decide on his activity regimen. Nurses must be careful, however, to make sure that the adolescent will still be getting sufficient exercise. A controversial article was recently published on this topic by Dr. Shelby Dietrich. In this article, Dr. Dietrich states " . . . that a competent physiotherapist can completely avoid repeated bleeding episodes and predicts that if today's hemophiliac children are maintained on active exercise therapy, in 20 or 30 years deformity will no longer be a consequence of hemarthrisis" (Dietrich, 1974). The exact amount of recommended exercise is still a point of contention, but there is now strong support for hemophiliacs remaining physically active. For the adolescent hemophiliac, such activities as swimming and golfing should be encouraged. The key to exercise is choosing the right activities with guidance from a physical therapist, physician, or nurse.

An area of preventing hemorrhages which is easier to control involves replacing the deficient factor before such procedures as dental work, surgery, or repeated intravenous or intramuscular injections. In general, surgery is contraindicated in the hemophiliac patient. If it is unavoidable, factor VIII levels must be increased preoperatively and for 10-14 days postoperatively (Aledort, 1977). A a result of the enormous risk that surgery incurs, good preventative care of the joints, teeth, and gums must be maintained. Joint bleeds should be treated promptly with factor replacements to prevent joint deformity and the possible need for reconstructive surgery. Both the adolescent and his family should be taught dental care by either the nurse or a dentist. This should include restriction of re-fined carbohydrates, ingestion of fluoride, periodic dental examina-tions, use of a soft-bristled toothbrush, regular flossing, and rinsing the mouth frequently to keep the oral cavity problem-free (Bittner, 1974). A final point to impress on the adolescent hemophiliac and his family is that health care should not consist solely of visits to the doctor during hemorrhages. It shuld be consistent and conscientious in both good times and bad.

Another area of patient teaching in pre-crisis is the frequently overlooked subject of diet. The parents and the adolescent himself should be aware of the need for a proper diet. Since adolescence is often a time of fad diets and junk food, reinforcement and monitoring of the diet may be necessary. The adolescent should be aware of the importance of limiting heavily spiced and other potentially ulcer-producing foods to decrease the chance of gastrointestinal bleeding. Parents should be aided in developing a diet plan for their adolescent hemophiliac that will provide all the essential nutrients without caus-ing obesity, which is harmful because it places further stress on joints and may in turn cause bleeding. Also, overweight patients need more concentrate to control hemorrhage (Bittner, 1974). If the nurse does not feel competent in diet counseling, then a referral to a nutritionist would be indicated.

Pre-crisis patient teaching on drugs is also fundamental to any nursing care plan. A common guideline for all hemophiliac patients and their families is to avoid aspirin or any drug that prolongs bleed-ing. The labels of all medications should be checked for aspirin con-tent before administering it. Acetaminophen is recommended as a substitute for aspirin. A pamphlet on pain control published by the National Hemophilia Foundation provides the following list of medica-tions to avoid: 1) Aspirin, 2) Butazolidin, 3) Phenacetin, 4) Indocin, and 5) Glyceryl guaiacolate, which is in Robitussin and Triaminic (Levine, 1975). Not all of these medications have been proven con-clusively to be harmful, but there is enough evidence to strongly sug-gest avoiding them. Nurses should be aware of these lists, inform their hemophiliac patients of their contents, and refer their patients to the National Hemophilia Foundation if they have any further ques-tions on this matter.

The next topic that requires patient teaching in the pre-crisis stage is that of providing a safe environment for the hemophiliac adolescent. A wealth of knowledge is available in the literature on establishing a safe environment for hemophiliac children, but when it comes to the adolescent there is very little. Most adolescents and their families have to rely on common sense as far as safety is concerned. This works relatively well for some families, but the nurse should assess the family's safety practices and make additional recommendations where they are needed. An article that appeared in Nursing 77 on safety practices for patients on anticoagulation therapy provides helpful suggestions for preventing accidents. These include using an electric shaver instead of a razor, using any sharp instrument carefully, avoiding the use of power tools, and instructions regarding nail and dental care (Moore & Maschak, 1977).

Some of the recommendations may seem so obvious that they do not need to be discussed, but, in reality, many hemophiliacs overlook these points. Therefore, a part of all patient teaching should be to remind the hemophiliac and his family of these considerations. It might also be of value to make a safety assessment of the home environment. Stairwells should be checked for railings and lighting, throw rugs (especially on hardwood floors) should be avoided, and seatbelts should be worn in the car at all times. Some of these suggestions may seem tedious, especially to the impulsive adolescent, but in terms of preventing bleeding crises, they are worth the effort.

Patient teaching in pre-crisis should also involve the hemophiliac's family. Hemophilia is disruptive and distressing to the family. The mother may feel guilty because she transmitted the disease. Siblings may be upset by the illness or jealous of the extra attention given to their brother (National Hemophilia Foundation, 1972). It is not possible for patient teaching to be successful if it is just focused on the hemophiliac. The entire family must be actively involved in the care and support of the afflicted member. A recent development in the care of the hemophiliac—home therapy— specifically addresses this need for active involvement. In this program, factor concentrates are kept in the home and patients and families are instructed on how to infuse them at the first sign of bleeding. Not only does the family become involved in his care, but so does the adolescent, who developmentally requires this independence and control. Home therapy provides an important opportunity to promote useful autonomy and independence for the patient and an improved life style for his family. It is becoming a common way to remedy the feelings of futility, guilt, and despair often experienced by the hemophiliac and his family (van Eys, 1977).

The professional nurse's role in home therapy is particularly important. Since this treatment modality is relatively new (1970), much patient teaching and education of health professionals is needed. Because of her experience and expertise, the nurse is the ideal person to make families aware of home therapy and to educate them about it. The nurse and physician's first responsibility is to determine eligibility. Generally, the criteria include such things as: "a confirmed diagnosis of hemophilia, emotional stability, ability to start intravenous injections, ability to prepare clotting factor, and a competent, supervisory physician" (van Eys, 1977, p. 5). There are also age limits on the program, "in the United States, the age limit has been set as low as four and as high as 12 years" (van Eys, 1977, p. 5). Usually, school-age children of around the age of nine years are the first to begin home therapy. This aids these patients in their developmental task of industry, which carries over into adolescence, creating a better-adjusted adolescent. Early reports suggest that home therapy may promote a normalization of life activities (Aledort, 1975). Additional benefits of home therapy include a more mobile life style for the family and earlier treatment of bleeding episodes. Hence, the hemophiliac and his family benefit socially (more traveling), psychologically (greater control), and physically (earlier treatment), from home therapy.

After the nurse has finished patient teaching on infusions, signs of bleeding, and preparation of factor VIII, the job is still not complete. A chart of when, why, and how much factor was used should be maintained. This chart should be reviewed at regular intervals when the patient comes in for examinations. In this way the nurse initiates, monitors, and maintains the home therapy program. Sufficient follow-up visits and reinforcement of teaching are important to assure the family that it is not being abandoned by the health care system. For more specific information on home therapy, the reader should consult the National Hemophilia Foundation's pamphlet, "Home Therapy for Hemophilia," and should use their videotapes, films, and cassettes as instructional materials. Home therapy is not the answer for every hemophiliac but, to the adolescent in particular, this opportunity for independence and control may provide the missing link for normal growth and development.

Finally, to conclude the pre-crisis stage, one last point needs to be mentioned. Regardless of how thoroughly patient teaching is performed, it is of limited value unless follow-up assessments of comprehension and retention are made. Patient teaching should be a continuing process of reinforcement and clarification. If the nurse does not feel comfortable with a particular area of teaching, referrals should be made to other members of the health care team. Only in this manner can pre-crisis teaching be maximally beneficial in preventing crises from occurring.

CRISIS

Despite the consistency of pre-crisis care, crises do occur. Physical, social, or psychological coping mechanisms fail and there is an increasing insult to the body. Usually, a crisis is equated with a bleeding episode in the hemophiliac. In actuality, however, other crises may occur such as joint deformities, pain, anemia, kidney malfunction, hepatitis, factor antibody formation, social isolation, and abnormal growth and development. If a crisis occurs, additional coping mechanisms must be instituted and nursing interventions must aim to advance the patient quickly to the post-crisis phase. In this section on crisis, a few major crises of hemophilia and their possible avenues of resolution will be explored. The reader is referred to the bibliography for additional information.

Before focusing on any particular crisis, however, the reason why coping mechanisms fail should be investigated. It is obvious from the extensive array of preventative measures discussed in the pre-crisis section that there are many crisis-provoking events for the hemophiliac adolescent. It is therefore understandable that some of these coping mechanisms will be insufficient at times to prevent a crisis. For example, bleeding into joints is sometimes unavoidable, even when treatment is begun promptly. Thus, part of the nursing care plan should be devoted to psychologically preparing the patient for failure of pre-crisis coping mechanisms and helping him through the crisis. Both the nurse and the patient must learn to accept the inevitability of occasional crises and learn not to view them as personal defeats. Crises can be growth-producing and rewarding when they are handled correctly and promptly. As patients experience repeated successful attempts at mastering bleeding episodes, they develop a more positive outlook (National Hemophilia Foundation, 1972).

The first crisis to be studied is that of a hemorrhagic episode. Usually stemming from trauma in the adolescent hemophiliac, a hemorrhagic crisis is certain to affect every hemophiliac during his lifetime. Hemorrhage endangers the hemophiliac in a variety of ways. He may go into shock from rapid blood loss or become anemic from slow bleeding. Vital structures may be damaged and/or chronic disability may result from joint deformities, contractures, or paralysis (National Hemophilia Foundation, 1972). In order to prevent death or severe deformity, evaluation and treatment must be initiated upon the first sign of hemorrhage.

During an acute major bleeding episode, several sequential laboratory determinations of hemoglobin and hematocrit are useful in determining the volume of blood loss (Boone, 1976). Once the extent of the bleed has been determined, additional resources for providing factor VIII can be gathered. If the hemorrhage was extensive, whole blood may be utilized to replace lost fluids. It is rarely used to raise factor VIII levels, however, because of the high risk of fluid overload.

At the present time, three substances are used to raise factor VIII levels without greatly expanding the circulating volume. These are: fresh frozen plasma from a donor who has very high amounts of factor VIII in the blood; cryoprecipitate, which is a factor VIII precipitate prepared relatively cheaply and readily from fresh frozen plasma; and commercial preparations. The latter may be more expensive than cryoprecipitate, and the hepatitis risk is higher than from single donor products (van Eys, 1977). The aim of therapy is to administer enough factor VIII to produce normal hemostasis. In most cases, simply utilizing these additional coping mechanisms—clotting factor solutions, rest, and ice packs—is enough to resolve the bleeding crisis. Nurses can reassure patients that the blood will be reabsorbed into the body in a few days and they will move into post-crisis.

In such hemorrhagic episodes as bleeding into a joint, however, further coping mechanisms and resources are necessary, including instruction for home care. After the pain and swelling subside, physical therapy may be ordered. Both the nurse and the physical therapist can instruct the adolescent hemophiliac of the plan of care so he can be in charge of his own care at home. In this way the adolescent can enjoy more independence and control. This intervention can be essential to the adolescent's social and psychological well-being because he will feel that he has more control over his own destiny. As long as these joint hemorrhages are treated promptly and are not too frequent, permanent damage should not result. If bleeding into the joint is prolonged or frequent, however, the need for orthopedic appliances or joint reconstruction may create additional crises (Boone & Spence, 1976).

An additional crisis stemming from the crisis of hemorrhage is that of hepatitis. Unfortunately, this potential crisis is difficult to control. Blood donors are screened for hepatitis, but the screening test is not 100 percent accurate (Liggins, 1976). Therefore, as far as the risk of hepatitis is concerned, there is little that can be done in the pre-crisis stage. It is more of a "wait and see" phenomenon that the hemophiliac may hope to avoid but must receive treatment for when the crisis occurs. The most important role of the nurse, then, is to assist the patient to view his problem, realistically, and as a temporary complication.

One last crisis that results from hemorrhagic episodes and factor replacement is the development of inhibitors or antibodies to the replacement factor. This occurs because the body begins producing proteins that destroy the infused factor VIII. Like hepatitis, this is difficult to predict or cope with in the pre-crisis stage. Inhibitors can occur and produce a crisis without warning. This is very difficult for the adolescent hemophiliac to accept while he is still struggling to adjust to his illness. The nurse must help him express his feelings of fear and frustration. Most distressing is the fact that no real solution to the crisis has yet been developed. Immunosuppressive drugs are under study but the results are inconclusive (Liggins, 1976). It is evident that additional coping mechanisms and resources need to be developed to resolve this crisis. In the meantime, the only way to deal with the problem is to have periodic antibody titers performed for early detection. The nurse should make sure that these titers are performed and also monitor the patient's response to the amounts of factor used for each bleeding episode. This crisis can occur at any age so all hemophiliac adolescents and their families should be prepared for this possibility.

Only the physical crises of hemophilia have been discussed so far. The complexities of this condition, however, can also cause significant social and psychological crises for the adolescent. An intricate psychological problem for the adolescent concerns overdependence and the inability to complete developmental tasks. Despite the preventative interventions in pre-crisis designed to involve the adolescent in his own care, adolescents sometimes become overdependent. If this situation is temporary, no crisis should result. If the adolescent remains this way, however, his developmental growth will become stagnant, and he will experience a crisis. "The imposition of a new need for dependence, superimposed on his earnest strivings for independence, may arouse frustration, anger, and ambivalence" (Tiedt, 1972). The adolescent may thus develop a negative self-concept as a result of his dependency feelings. He may feel that he will never be able to function on his own, and he may enter into post-crisis and maladptation.

Nurses must always encourage independence in adolescent hemophiliacs. Transient periods of regression and dependence are normal, but if the adolescent enters a crisis with chronic dependence additional resources will be needed. While the nurse must be supportive of the adolescent in a dependency crisis, early efforts must be made to encourage independence. Small attempts at self-reliance by the adolescent should be recognized by the nurse and praised. The family also should be taught to allow the adolescent to help himself and to not always anticipate his needs. Lastly, however, if the adolescent becomes chronically dependent, a psychiatric referral is indicated.

A final crisis to be discussed is social in nature. This is the crisis of undereducation. Due to the nature of hemophilia and its requirement for hospitalizations or rest at home, absenteeism from school is a major problem. This factor poses a significant crisis to the adolescent hemophiliac. Not only will undereducation affect his social relationships and self-concept, it will also decrease his job opportunities. A survey of adult hemophiliacs found a 27 percent unemployment rate with 19 percent chronically unemployed (Weiss, 1977).

It is easy to see the spiral of social crises leading to psychological and physical crises. The adolescent who misses school is unable to graduate, unable to find a job, unable to support a family, unable to afford proper medical treatment and so on. Therefore, a holistic approach to care cannot be overemphasized. All aspects of the adolescent hemophiliac's life must be attended to. Such additional resources as tutors should be utilized when the adolescent must miss school. If this is not possible, then social workers can be invaluable in obtaining school assignments for the adolescent. A few minutes spent on resolving a crisis of forced absenteeism from school can prevent many future crises of unemployment, poverty, and psychological anguish (Tiedt, 1972).

In summary, this section illustrated the additional coping mechanisms, resources, psychosocial support, and nursing interventions needed to care for the adolescent hemophiliac in crisis. Each of these areas was addressed in the context of a particular physical, psychological, or social crisis. In each case, interventions were suggested that could aid the client in realistically viewing his problem and in limiting the severity of his crisis. It is hoped that, by mobilizing these recommended additional resources and coping mechanisms, the hemophiliac adolescent can expediently progress to post-crisis.

POST-CRISIS

Once the preventative measures of pre-crisis have failed and the additional resources of crisis have been mobilized, the hemophiliac adolescent enters the stage of post-crisis. In this stage, two outcomes are possible. The first is a maximum level of wellness in which physically, socially, and/or psychologically the hemophiliac attains the highest potential of growth after the crisis. The second is destruction, or maladaptation, where the crisis has resulted in a physically, socially, and/or psychologically lower state than the hemophiliac was in during pre-crisis. Both of these possibilities will be analyzed in depth with specific examples of both. Also, the particular nursing interventions most applicable to both of these outcomes will be addressed.

The first point to be made is that hemophilia is a condition which frequently and chronically runs the course from pre-crisis through post-crisis. It is a pattern of exacerbations, rehabilitations, and remissions. Rehabilitation of hemophiliac patients is a life-long process because acute problems become chronic manifestations. Thus, post-crisis is an important stage to focus on, since rehabilitation and readjustment to changes imposed by hemophilia become a way of life. No problem in hemophilia can ever be viewed as an isolated incident; it must always be looked at in terms of its long-range consequences. "The momentary success of stopping a bleed is a Pyrrhic victory if, at the age of 25, he's a cripple, confined to a wheelchair or braces" (Liggins, 1976). All nursing interventions after the crisis stage must therefore concentrate on working towards and maintaining the client at a maximum level of wellness. If this is not successful, then the second alternative of maladaptation will become a reality.

The alternative of the maximum level of wellness will be analyzed first. For the hemophiliac adolescent, fortunately, the maximum level of wellness is the usual outcome of a physical crisis. The bleeding episodes discussed in the section on crisis, for example, are usually quickly resolved in the adolescent hemophiliac by the infusion of a factor concentrate. As long as the bleed does not extensively involve a joint and is treated promptly, total recovery with a minimum of post-crisis stage rehabilitation is the norm. A few days of rest and physical therapy may be required but permanent damage is usually alleviated. Therefore, if pre-crisis teaching on the signs and symptoms of a bleed and crisis stage factor therapy have been successful, then the post-crisis stage should also have a positive result. Additional nursing interventions in the post-crisis stage, after a bleed, are summed up as follows: "After all bleeding episodes . . . watch closely for signs of further bleeding, such as increased pain and swelling, fever, or symptoms of shock. Closely monitor PTT, if less than 100 seconds, clotting factor levels are sufficient" (Dressler, 1980). Finally, the nurse should also reinforce the pre-crisis teaching that was done and give recognition to the adolescent's accomplishments.

Similar to physical crises, social and psychological crises can also result in a maximum level of wellness in post-crisis. The key to success with these emotional crises seems to be directly dependent on the support that the adolescent hemophiliac receives from his family and the health care team. "The ideal behavioral response . . . is the development of an active, independent state that is sought by the hemophiliac and supported or promoted by his family and physicians" (Green, 1976). If, for example, the crisis had been an overdependence or problems with social relationships and school, a positive post-crisis outcome could be attainable with family and professional support. The most important factor to keep in mind in post-crisis is that we professionals must augment the adolescent hemophiliac's capabilities. As the adolescent hemophiliac emerges from a crisis of overdependence, for example, nurses must take the time to review this experience with him and encourage him to talk about his plans, his successes, and his failures (Tiedt, 1972). The nurse must also remember that the accomplishment of independence is a great achievement for the adolescent hemophiliac and should acknowledge it appropriately.

Another indicator of a positive outcome in post-crisis is the adolescent's successful attainment of a healthy activity regime. As mentioned earlier, an illustration of a negative outcome in activity levels in the adolescent hemophiliac is risk taking, although some risk-taking behavior is essential. Often, if the family has been too restrictive, or the adolescent has been unable to cope with his disease, he may resort to denial or self-destructive activities. Most adolescents do eventually find a balance in their lives between risk taking and a satisfying life style. An absolute restriction in activity may not always be the healthiest program. Rather, a moderation of some risk-taking behavior with a sensible activity scheme may be more psychologically healthy.

An example of some advancement in this area is the idea of summer camps for hemophiliacs—these were formed to allow the hemophiliac child or adolescent to have a more normal life style. Activities are kept as normal as possible but modified to lower the risk of bleeding. In this way, the campers are allowed to practice some risky activities under supervision and care (Boutaugh & Patterson, 1977).

It should thus be a major nursing intervention in post-crisis to evaluate the amounts and types of activities that the hemophiliac has chosen to determine if they are truly healthy. If the nurse feels that an activity regimen is not safe, she may have to risk creating a new crisis for the adolescent by helping him to revise his plan. This may be difficult, but the benefits in the long run will far outweigh the short-term liabilities.

We will now analyze the unsuccessful conclusion in post-crisis— maladaptation. In this situation, the resolution of the crisis has not resulted in growth but, rather, in disarray. An example of malad- aptation to a physical crisis is that of a joint bleed leading to a per- manent deformity. This is a perfect example of the pre-crisis and crisis resources failing and the client emerging in post-crisis at a chronically lower level of functioning. Joint bleeding can lead to or- thopedic problems (Liggins, 1976). Once this chronically debilitating and destructive process begins in the joint, little can be done to ar- rest it. Further care should concentrate on trying to slow down the progress of the deterioration of the joint. The main treatment at this point is physical therapy to maintain mobility and strength in the affected part.

In this situation, the nurse can be instrumental in ensuring that the patient's care is holistic and does not just focus on the problem joint (Boone, 1976). Although the hemophiliac's joint condition will not be greatly improved or cured, a positive outlook can be main- tained by strengthening the rest of the body. This attitude should be stressed with the adolescent whose body image might be seriously damaged by this complication. To compensate, the nurse and the physical therapist should help the patient and his family to focus on the healthy parts of his body.

The last area to be explored is that of psychological and social maladaptation. As stated previously, many adolescent hemophiliacs resolve their emotional crises well. This is due mainly to the sup- port that they receive from their family and the health team. For adolescent hemophiliacs who may not have these supports, however, the stresses of the disease may be too great. Instead of openly ex- pressing anxiety and experiencing growth, the adolescent may chan- nel his anxiety into such maladaptive behaviors as bossiness and attempts to control others (Hilgartner, 1976). The greatest contribution that the nurse can make in this situation is to work with the family and other professionals in uncovering the root cause of the anxiety. Maladaptive behaviors should be looked at as a clue to the underlying problem and not the problem itself. Hence, the major nursing interventions that should be utilized are those of support and understanding of the adolescent, and aiding him to verbalize his feelings and perceive the situation realistically.

The family of the adolescent hemophiliac can also experience maladaptive behaviors. After the medical crisis is past, parents may feel depressed, irritable, and useless. It often helps parents to discuss these feelings (National Hemophilia Foundation, 1972). Therefore, the post-crisis nursing care plan must address the need of the hemophiliac's family after a crisis. Nurses must keep in mind that a crisis affects the entire realm of significant others as well as the adolescent. Nursing interventions utilized to aid the adolescent hemophiliac during maladaptation should thus also be applied to his family. Post-crisis, perhaps more than any other stage, requires a team effort to support the patient and his family in their positive or negative outcome.

CONCLUSIONS

It has been the goal of this chapter to illustrate how the crisis theory model can be utilized to structure nursing care for such a complex chronic disease as hemophilia. Crisis theory enables the nurse to holistically view the physical, social, and psychological ramifications of this disease. Judging from the myriad of interventions listed in this chapter, it is evident that one professional alone cannot provide comprehensive care to the hemophiliac. Thus, it is crucial that a team of health professionals from varying areas of expertise be assembled to work together for the benefit of the patient. Interdisciplinary teams which include the patient and his family are the key to successful treatment and continued growth and development.

The content of this chapter is unique in that it is one of the first works to combine developmental theory, holistic care, crisis theory, and hemophilia into one composite. This is by no means an end in itself, however. Research is still needed in the area of teaching interventions, preventative measures for hemophiliacs, and supportive efforts for adolescent hemophiliacs and their families. Also, further research into the genetics of hemophilia and new treatment for hemophiliacs needs to be conducted. Nurses can contribute to the improvement of care for adolescent hemophiliacs by conducting further studies in the area of holistic care and by implementing this approach in their practice. The literature is seriously lacking in material on adolescent hemophilia and on hemophilia in general. As professional nurses we should either contribute to or assist in the advancement of publication in this area.

BIBLIOGRAPHY ON HEMOPHILIA

Aledort, L. M. Current management: A physician's manual. New York: National Hemophilia Foundation, 1978.

Aledort, L. M. The management of hemophilia. Drug Therapy, The Mount Sinai School of Medicine, 1971, 1(3), 1-4.

Aledort, L. M. (Ed.). Recent advances in hemophilia. New York: The New York Academy of Sciences, 1975.

Aledort, L. M., & Levine, P. H. Surgery in hemophilia. New York: National Hemophilia Foundation, 1977.

Batz, H. A new life for Artie. Hartford Courant, Feb. 17, 1974.

Bittner, E. F. Your child and hemophilia. A manual for parents. Los Angeles: Orthopedic Hospital, 1974 (distributed by National Hemophilia Foundation, 1975).

Boone, D. C. (Ed.). Comprehensive management of hemophilia. Philadelphia: F. A. Davis Co., 1976.

Boone, D. C., & Spence, C. D. Physical therapy in hemophilia. New York: The National Hemophilia Foundation, 1976.

Boutaugh, M., & Patterson, P. C. Summer camp for hemophiliacs. American Journal of Nursing, 1977, 77, 1288-1291.

Brinkhous, K. M., & Hemker, H. C. Handbook of hemophilia. New York: American Elsevier Publishing Co., Inc., 1975.

Dietrich, S. L. New prescription for hemophilia: Exercise. Medical World News, May 3, 1974.

Dietrich, S. L. Hemophilia, a total approach to treatment and rehabilitation. Los Angeles: Orthopedic Hospital, 1968.

Dietrich, S. L. Comprehensive care for the person with hemophilia. New York: National Hemophilia Foundation, 1977.

Dressler, D. Understanding and treating hemophilia. Nursing 80, Aug. 1980, 72-73.

Erikson, E. H. (Ed.). The challenge of youth. New York: Anchor Books, 1963.

Garlinghouse, J., & Sharp, L. J. Self-concept and family stress in relation to bleeding episodes. Nursing Research, Jan.-Feb. 1968, 32-37.

Green, D. (Ed.). Hemophilia. Springfield, Ill.: Charles C. Thomas, 1976.

Having hemophilia. Medical World News, July 25, 1977.

Hilgartner, M. W. (Ed.). Hemophilia in children. Littleton, Mass.: Publishing Sciences Group, 1976.

Improved odds: A prenatal test for hemophilia. Time, May 14, 1979, p. 107.

Levine, P. H. Control for pain in hemophilia. New York: National Hemophilia Foundation, 1975.

Liggins, M. R. (Ed.). When hemophilia heads the problem list. Patient Care, Oct. 15, 1976, 58-83.

Moore, K., & Maschak, B. How patient education can reduce the risks of anticoagulation. Nursing 77, Sept. 1977, 24-29.

The National Hemophilia Foundation. Psychological aspects of hemophilia. New York: The National Hemophilia Foundation, 1972.

The National Hemophilia Foundation. The hemophilic child in school. New York: The National Hemophilia Foundation, 1974.

Rhinelander, D. H. Fetus test near for hemophilia. Hartford Courant, April 26, 1978.

Rice, P. F. The adolescent. Boston: Allyn and Bacon, 1978.

Ross, J. K. E. A boy with hemophilia. Nursing Times, Nov. 15, 1979, 1972-1974.

A saving factor for hemophiliacs. Medical World News, March 1, 1974.

Seidman, J. M. (Ed.). The adolescent. New York: Holt, Rinehart and Winston, 1960.

Strauss, H. S. Diagnosis and treatment of hemophilia. New York: Herbert S. Strauss, 1972.

Tiedt, E. The adolescent in the hospital. Nursing Forum, 1972, 11(2), 120-140.

van Eys, J. (Ed.). Home therapy for hemophilia. New York: The National Hemophilia Foundation, 1977.

Weiss, A. E. Modern management of hemophilia. Resident and Staff Physician, Sept. 1977, 74-87.

References

Abdellah, F. G., et al. Patient-centered approaches to nursing.
New York: Macmillan Co., 1960.
Aguilera, D. C., & Messick, J. M. Crisis intervention: Theory
and methodology. St. Louis: C. V. Mosby Co., 1970.
Alicine, A. Crisis theory conceptual framework. Unpublished term
paper, University of Connecticut School of Nursing, 1980.
Auger, J. R. Behavioral systems and nursing. Englewood Cliffs,
N.J.: Prentice-Hall, 1976.
Bain, P. T., Hales, L. W., & Rand, L. P. An investigation of
some assumptions and characteristics of the pass/fail grading
system. The Journal of Educational Research, 1973, 67(3),
134-136.
Barrell, L. M. Crisis intervention: Partnership in problem-
solving. Nursing Clinics of North America, 1974, 9, 5-16.
Beckstrand, J. The notion of a practice theory and the relationship
of scientific and ethical knowledge to practice. Research in
Nursing and Health, 1978, 1, 131-136.
Benedek, T. Parenthood as a developmental phase. A contribution
to the libido theory. Journal of the American Psychoanalytic
Association, 1959, 7, 389-417.
Bennis, W., Benne, K. D., Chin, R., & Corey, K. E. The Planning of Change (3rd ed.). New York: Holt, Rinehart & Winston,
1976.
Bigge, M. L. Learning theories for teachers. New York: Harper
and Row, 1976.

Bloom, B. S. (Ed.). Taxonomy of educational objectives, Handbook I: Cognitive domain. New York: David McKay Co., 1956.

Bloom, B. S. Definitional aspects of the crisis concept. Journal of Consulting Psychology, 1963, 27, 498-502.

Bobbitt, F. The curriculum. Boston: Houghton Mifflin Co., 1918.

Bobbitt, F. How to make a curriculum. Boston: Houghton Mifflin Co., 1924.

Bode, B. H. How we learn. Boston: D. C. Heath and Co., 1940.

Bridgman, M. Collegiate education for nursing. New York: Russell Sage Foundation, 1953.

Broncatello, K. F. Auger in action: Application of the model. Advances in Nursing Science, 1980, 2(2), 13-23.

Brown, D. L. Curriculum project evaluation report (classes of 1971-1978). Unpublished report, Storrs, Conn.: University of Connecticut School of Nursing, 1979.

Brown, D. L. Curriculum project evaluation report addendum. Unpublished report, Storrs, Conn.: University of Connecticut School of Nursing, 1981.

Brown, E. L. Nursing for the future. New York: Russell Sage Foundation, 1948.

Bruner, J. The process of education. Cambridge: Harvard University Press, 1960.

Bruton, M. The process of curriculum revision. Nursing Outlook, 1974, 22, 310-314.

Burr, W. R. Theory construction and the sociology of the family. New York: John Wiley & Sons, Inc., 1973.

Bush, H. A. Models for nursing. Advances in Nursing Science, 1979, 1(2), 13-21.

Caplan, G. An approach to community mental health. New York: Grune and Stratton, 1961.

Caplan, G. Principles of preventive psychiatry. New York: Basic Books, 1964.

Caplan, G. A public health approach to child psychiatry. Mental Hygiene, 1951, 35, 235-249.

Caplan, G., Mason, E., & Kaplan, D. Four studies of crisis in parents of prematures. Community Mental Health Journal, 1965, 1, 149-161.

Carper, B. A. Fundamental patterns of knowing in nursing. Advances in Nursing Science, 1978, 1(1), 13-23.

Caswell, H. L. Emergence of the curriculum as a field of professional work and study. In H. F. Robison (Ed.), Precedents and promise in the curriculum field. New York: Teacher's College Press, 1966.

Caswell, H. L., & Campbell, D. S. Curriculum development. New York: American Book Co., 1935.

Charters, W. W. Curriculum construction. New York: Macmillan Co., 1923.

Chater, S. S. A conceptual framework for curriculum development. Nursing Outlook, 1975, 23, 428-433.

Chater, S., Kramer, M., & Tone, D. Nursing Research, a videotape series developed by Cooperative Graduate Education in Nursing, American Journal of Nursing Co., New York, 1975.

Chin, R. The utility of systems models and developmental models for practitioners. In J. P. Riehl & C. Roy (Eds.), Conceptual models for nursing practice (2nd ed.). New York: Appleton-Century-Crofts, 1980, 21-37.

Commission on Sex Bias in Measurement. AMEG commission report on sex bias in interest measurement. Measurement and Evaluation in Guidance, 1973, 6(3), 171-177.

Committee on the Function of Nursing. A program for the nursing profession. New York: Macmillan Co., 1948.

Committee on the Grading of Nursing Schools. Nursing schools today and tomorrow. New York: Committee on the Grading of Nursing Schools, 1934.

Conley, V. C. Curriculum and instruction in nursing. Boston: Little, Brown and Co., 1973.

D'Amato, C. Crisis intervention during the puerperium: An empirical test of a nursing intervention. Unpublished term paper, University of Connecticut School of Nursing, 1978.

Darbonne, A. Crisis: A review of theory, practice and research. International Journal of Psychiatry, 1968, 6, 371-379.

Davis, F., Oleson, V., & Whittaker, E. W. Problems and issues in collegiate nursing education. In F. Davis (Ed.), The nursing profession: Five sociological essays. New York: John Wiley & Sons, 1966.

Department of Baccalaureate and Higher Degree Programs. Faculty-curriculum development, part I, The process of curriculum development. New York: National League for Nursing, 1974a.

Department of Baccalaureate and Higher Degree Programs. Faculty-curriculum development, part II, Curriculum evaluation. New York: National League for Nursing, 1974b.

Department of Baccalaureate and Higher Degree Programs. Faculty-curriculum development, part III, Conceptual framework—Its meaning and function. New York: National League for Nursing, 1975a.

Department of Baccalaureate and Higher Degree Programs. Faculty-curriculum development, part IV, Unifying the curriculum—The integrated approach. New York: National League for Nursing, 1974c.

Department of Baccalaureate and Higher Degree Programs. Faculty-curriculum development, part V, The changing role of the professional nurse—Implications for nursing education. New York: National League for Nursing, 1975b.

Department of Baccalaureate and Higher Degree Programs. Faculty-curriculum development, part VI, Curriculum revision in baccalaureate nursing education. New York: National League for Nursing, 1975c.

Department of Services to Schools, National League of Nursing Education. Nursing organization curriculum conference, Curriculum Bulletin, No. 1. New York: National League of Nursing Education, 1950.

Department of Services to Schools, National League of Nursing Education. Joint nursing curriculum conference, Curriculum Bulletin, No. 2. New York: National League of Nursing Education, 1951.

DeTornyay, R. Strategies for teaching nursing. New York: John Wiley & Sons, 1971.

Dewey, J. Democracy and education. New York: The Free Press, 1966. (Original edition published by Macmillan Company, 1916.)

Dickoff, J., & James, P. A theory of theories: A position paper. Nursing Research, 1968, 17, 197–203.

Dock, L. A short history of nursing. New York: G. P. Putnam's Sons, 1920.

Dolan, J. A. Nursing in society (14th ed.). Philadelphia: W. B. Saunders Co., 1978.

Donaldson, S. K., & Crowley, D. M. The discipline of nursing. Nursing Outlook, 1978, 26, 113–120.

Doob, L. W. Eidetic images among the Ibo. Ethnology, 1964, 3, 357–363.

Downs, F. S. Clinical and theoretical research. In F. S. Downs & J. W. Fleming (Eds.), Issues in nursing research. New York: Appleton-Century-Crofts, 1979.

Duffey, M., & Muhlenkamp, A. F. A framework for theory analysis. Nursing Outlook, 1974, 22, 570–574.

Dunn, H. A. High-level wellness for man and society. American Journal of Public Health, 1959, 49(6), 786–792.

Dyer, E. D. Parenthood as crisis: A re-study. Marriage and Family Living, 1963, 25, 196-201.

Elliott, F. Viewpoints on curriculum development. New York: National League for Nursing, 1957.

Ellis, R. Characteristics of significant theories. Nursing Research, 1968, 17, 217-222.

Erikson, E. H. Childhood and society (2nd ed.). New York: Norton, 1963.

Fagan, E. A. Accreditation as I see it. Nursing Outlook, 1960, 8(1), 41-43.

Fawcett, J. Body image and the pregnant couple. MCN, The American Journal of Maternal Child Nursing, 1978b, 3, 227-233.

Fawcett, J. The relationship between identification and patterns of change in spouses' body images during and after pregnancy. International Journal of Nursing Studies, 1977, 14, 199-213.

Fawcett, J. The Roy adaptation model: A framework for assessing and understanding the cesarean father. In C. F. Kehoe (Ed.), The cesarean experience: Theoretical and clinical perspectives for nurses. New York: Appleton-Century-Crofts, 1981.

Fawcett, J. The "what" of theory development. In Theory development: What, why, how? New York: National League for Nursing, 1978a.

Flexner, A. Medical education in the United States and Canada. Boston: D. B. Updike, The Merrymount Press, 1910.

Gage, N. L. Paradigms for research on teaching. In N. L. Gage (Ed.), Handbook of research on teaching. Chicago: Rand McNally, 1963.

Gagne, R. M. The conditions of learning. New York: Holt, Rinehart and Winston, 1970.

Goldmark, J. Nursing and nursing education in the United States. Report of the Committee for the Study of Nursing Education and Report of a Survey by Josephine Goldmark. New York: Macmillan Co., 1923.

Goodlad, J. Curriculum: A Janus look. The Record, 1968, 70, 95-107.

Goodlad, J. I., & Richter, M. N. The development of a conceptual system for dealing with problems of curriculum and instruction, Cooperative Research Project No. 454. Los Angeles: University of California and Institute for Development of Educational Activities, 1966.

Goodwin, B. An investigation of the relationship between psychoprophylaxis in childbirth and changes in concept of self and concept of husband (Doctoral dissertation, New York University, 1970). Dissertation Abstracts International, 1971, 31:11:6714B.

Gordon, M., & Anello, M. A systematic approach to curriculum revision. Nursing Outlook, 1974, 22, 306-310.

Gough, H. G. California psychological inventory manual. Palo Alto, Cal.: Consulting Psychologists Press, 1969.

Gray, J. Education for nursing. Minneapolis: University of Minnesota Press, 1960.

Green, J., & Stone, J. C. Curriculum evaluation theory and practice. New York: Springer, 1977.

Greer, G. D., Jr., Hitt, J. D., Sitterley, T. E., & Slobodnick, S. B. An examination of four major factors impacting on psychomotor performance effectiveness. In The psychomotor domain. A resource book for media specialists. Washington, D.C.: Gryphon House, 1972.

Gronlund, N. E. Stating behavioral objectives for classroom instruction. New York: Macmillan Co., 1970.

Haber, R. Eidetic images. Scientific American, 1969, 36-44.

Hagemeier, D., & Hunt, C. Do new graduates use conceptual framework? Nursing Outlook, 1979, 27, 545-548.

Hales, L. W., Bain, P. T., & Rand, L. P. The pass fail system: The congruence between the rationale for and student reasons in election. The Journal of Educational Research, 1973, 66(7), 296.

Hall, K. V. Current trends in the use of conceptual frameworks in nursing education. Journal of Nursing Education, 1979, 18(4), 26-29.

Halpern, H. Crisis theory: A definitional study. Community Mental Health Journal, 1973, 9, 342-349.

Halpern, H. The crisis scale: A factor analysis and revision. Community Mental Health Journal, 1975, 11, 295-300.

Hardy, M. E. Theories: Components, development, and evaluation. Nursing Research, 1974, 23, 100-107.

Hardy, M. E. Evaluating nursing theory. In Theory development: What, why, how? New York: National League for Nursing, 1978.

Harrington, C. Experience with pass/not pass grading: Student views. Journal of College Student Personnel, 1974, 15(5), 379.

Harrow, A. J. A taxonomy of the psychomotor domain: A guide for developing behavioral objectives. New York: David McKay Co., 1972.

Havighurst, R. Developmental tasks and education (3rd ed.). New York: David McKay Co., 1972.

Hayes, E. Prediction of academic performance in a baccalaureate nursing program. Journal of Nursing Education, 1981, 20(6), 4-8.

Heidgerken, L. When is a course integrated? Nursing Outlook, 1955, 3(3), 128-129.

Heineman, D. Description of the setting. University of Connecticut School of Nursing Curriculum project report, academic year 1972-1973. Unpublished report. Storrs, Conn.: University of Connecticut School of Nursing, 1973.

Hilgard, E. R., & Bower, G. H. Theories of learning. New York: Appleton-Century-Crofts, 1966.

Hobbs, D. F., Jr. Parenthood as crisis: A third study. Journal of Marriage and the Family, 1965, 27, 357-362.

Hobbs, D. F., Jr., & Cole, S. P. Transition to parenthood: A decade replication. Journal of Marriage and the Family, 1976, 38, 723-731.

Hobbs, D. F., Jr., & Wimbish, J. M. Transition to parenthood by black couples. Journal of Marriage and the Family, 1977, 39, 677-688.

Homans, G. C. Bringing men back in. American Sociological Review, 1964, 29, 809-818.

Hott, J. An investigation of the relationship between psychoprophylaxis in childbirth and changes in self-concept of the participant husband and his concept of his wife. Image, 1972, 5(2), 11-15.

Huebner, D. The moribund curriculum field: Its wake and our work. Curriculum Inquiry, 1976, 6(2), 153-167.

Hunt, J. Intelligence and experience. New York: Ronald Press, 1961.

Infante, M. S. The clinical laboratory in nursing education. New York: John Wiley & Sons, 1975a.

Infante, M. S. A rationale for general education in nursing curricula. Journal of Nursing Education, 1975b, 14, 27-38.

Johnson, D. E. Development of theory: A requisite for nursing as a primary health profession. Nursing Research, 1974, 23, 372-377.

Johnson, D. E. The behavioral system model for nursing. In J. P. Riehl & C. Roy, Conceptual models for nursing practice (2nd ed.). New York: Appleton-Century-Crofts, 1980.

Johnson, W. R. The measurement and evaluation of student and faculty perceptions of nursing education environments: A summary report. An abstract for action: Appendices. New York: McGraw-Hill, 1971.

Kalisch, P. A., & Kalisch, B. J. The advance of American nursing. Boston: Little, Brown and Co., 1978.

Kelley, J. The conceptual framework in nursing education. In Faculty-curriculum development, part VI—Curriculum revision in baccalaureate nursing education. New York: National League for Nursing, 1975.

Kennedy, M. J., & Collins, J. Concepts of man. Paper presented to the Faculty of the University of Connecticut School of Nursing, Storrs, Conn., December 1974.

Kerlinger, F. N. Behavioral research. A conceptual approach. New York: Holt, Rinehart and Winston, 1979.

Kerlinger, F. N. Foundations of behavioral research (2nd ed.). New York: Holt, Rinehart and Winston, 1973.

King, I. M. A theory for nursing. Systems, concepts, process. New York: Wiley, 1981.

Kliebard, H. The curriculum field in retrospect. In P. W. F. Witt (Ed.), Technology and the curriculum. New York: Teacher's College Press, 1968.

Kliebard, H. M. Curriculum past and curriculum present. Educational Leadership, 1976, 33(1), 245-248.

Knowles, M. The modern practice of adult education. New York: Association Press, 1976.

Koehne, N., & Fawcett, J. Discussion of crisis theory. Paper presented to the Faculty of the University of Connecticut School of Nursing, May 1972.

Koehne, N., & Fawcett, J. The use of crisis theory as a conceptual framework for curriculum development. University of Connecticut School of Nursing. Unpublished memoranda, 1971-1972.

Kramer, M. Reality shock. St. Louis: C. V. Mosby Co., 1974.

Krathwohl, D. R., Bloom, B. S., & Masia, B. B. Taxonomy of educational objectives, handbook II: Affective domain. New York: David McKay Co., 1964.

Langford, T., Stephenson, J., & Stanley, T. Criteria for choosing textbooks for the nontraditional professional nursing curriculum. Journal of Nursing Education, 1973, 12(3), 2-8.

LeMasters, E. E. Parenthood as crisis. Marriage and Family Living, 1957, 19, 352-355.

Lindemann, E. The meaning of crisis in individual and family living. Teachers College Record, 1956, 57, 310-315.

Lindemann, E. Symptomatology and management of acute grief. American Journal of Psychiatry, 1944, 101, 141-148.

Litwack, L., Sakata, R., & Wykle, M. Counseling evaluation and student evaluation in nursing education. New York: Saunders, 1972.

Longway, I. M. Curriculum concepts—An historical analysis. Nursing Outlook, 1972, 20(2), 116-120.

MacDonald, G. Development of standards and accreditation in collegiate nursing education. New York: Teacher's College Press, 1965.

Mager, R. F. Preparing instructional objectives. Belmont, Cal.: Fearon Publishers, 1962.

Marut, J. S., & Mercer, R. T. Comparison of primiparas' perceptions of vaginal and cesarean births. Nursing Research, 1979, 28, 260-266.

McGillicuddy, M. C. A study of the relationship between mothers' rooming-in during their children's hospitalization and change in selected areas of children's behavior. In F. S. Downs & M. A. Newman (Eds.), A source book of nursing research (2nd ed.). Philadelphia: F. A. Davis, 1977.

McKay, R. P. The conceptual framework as a component of curriculum development. In Faculty-curriculum development, part III, Conceptual framework—Its meaning and function. New York: National League for Nursing, 1975.

McMurry, F. M. Some recollections of the past forty years of education. Peabody Journal of Education, 1927, 4, 325-332.

Merton, R. K. Social theory and social structure (Rev. ed.). New York: The Free Press, 1957.

Moloney, M. The integrated baccalaureate curriculum: An opinion survey. Nursing Outlook, 1978, 26, 375-379.

Murdock, J. E. Regrouping for an integrated curriculum. Nursing Outlook, 1978, 26, 514-519.

Murphy, E. An examination of crisis theory. Unpublished term paper, Boston University School of Nursing, 1980.

National League for Nursing, Department of Baccalaureate and Higher Degree Programs. Criteria for the appraisal of baccalaureate and higher degree programs in nursing. New York: National League for Nursing, 1972.

National League for Nursing, Department of Baccalaureate and Higher Degree Programs. Criteria for the appraisal of baccalaureate and higher degree programs in nursing. New York: National League for Nursing, 1977.

National League of Nursing Education. A curriculum guide for schools of nursing. New York: National League of Nursing Education, 1937.

National League of Nursing Education. Curriculum for schools of nursing. New York: National League of Nursing Education, 1927.

National League of Nursing Education. Essentials of a good school of nursing. New York: National League of Nursing Education, 1936a.

National League of Nursing Education. Manual of the essentials of a good hospital nursing service. New York: National League of Nursing Education, 1936b.

National League of Nursing Education. The nursing school faculty— Duties, qualities and preparation of its members. New York: National League of Nursing Education, 1933.

National League of Nursing Education. Standard curriculum for schools of nursing. New York: National League of Nursing Education, 1917.

Nursing Development Conference Group. Concept formalization in nursing: Process and product (2nd ed.). Boston: Little, Brown and Co., 1979.

Nursing Theories Conference Group. Nursing theories. Englewood Cliffs, N.J.: Prentice-Hall, 1980.

Nutting, M. A. Some ideals for schools of nursing. In M. A. Nutting (Ed.), A sound economic basis for schools of nursing. New York: G. P. Putnam's Sons, 1926.

Nye, F. I., & Berardo, F. M. Emerging conceptual frameworks in family analysis. New York: Macmillan Co., 1966.

Orem, D. E. Nursing: Concepts of practice (2nd ed.). New York: McGraw-Hill, 1980.

Ozimek, D. Accreditation of baccalaureate and masters degree programs in nursing. New York: National League for Nursing, 1974.

Palmer, M. E. Method of determining grades for clinical performance. Nursing Outlook, 1959, 7, 468-470.

Palmer, M. E. Self-evaluation of nursing performance based on clinical practice objectives. Boston: Boston University Press, 1962.

Palmer, M. E., & Woolley, A. The long and tortured history of clinical evaluation. Nursing Outlook, 1977, 25(5), 308-315.

Parad, H. Crisis intervention. New York: Family Service Association of America, 1965.

Parad, H., & Caplan, G. A. A framework for studying families in crisis. In H. Parad (Ed.), Crisis intervention. New York: Family Service Association of America, 1965.

Payton, O. D. Research: The validation of clinical practice. Philadelphia: F. A. Davis, 1979.

Peterson, C. J. Questions frequently asked about the development of a conceptual framework. Journal of Nursing Education, 1977, 16(4), 22-32.

Phenix, P. Realms of meaning. New York: McGraw-Hill, 1964.

Pittenger, O. E., & Gooding, C. T. Learning theories in educational practice. An integration of psychological theory and educational philosophy. New York: John Wiley & Sons, Inc., 1971.

Rapaport, L. The state of crisis: Some theoretical considerations. In H. Parad (Ed.), Crisis intervention. New York: Family Service of America, 1965.

Redman, B. The process of patient teaching in nursing. St. Louis: C. V. Mosby Co., 1972.

Redman, B. K. Why develop a conceptual framework? Journal of Nursing Education, 1974, 13(3), 2-10.

Reese, H. W., & Overton, W. F. Models of development and theories of development. In L. R. Goulet & P. B. Baltes (Eds.), Life-span developmental psychology. New York: Academic Press, 1970.

Reilly, D. E. Why a conceptual framework? Nursing Outlook, 1975, 23, 566-569.

Richards, M. Instructional technology: Problems and Prospects. Educational Forum, 1974, 38, 480-482.

Riehl, J. P., & Roy, C., Sr. Conceptual models for nursing practice (2nd ed.). New York: Appleton-Century-Crofts, 1980.

Riehl, J. P. Nursing models in current use. In J. P. Riehl & C. Roy, Conceptual models for nursing practice (2nd ed.). New York: Appleton-Century-Crofts, 1980.

Robischon, P. The challenge of crisis theory for nursing. Nursing Outlook, 1967, 15(7), 28-32.

Rogers, C. Freedom to learn. Columbus, Ohio: Charles E. Merrill Co., 1969.

Rogers, C. G. Conceptual models as guides to clinical nursing specialization. Journal of Nursing Education, 1973, 12(4), 2-6.

Rogers, C. G. Why develop a conceptual framework. Journal of Nursing Education, 1974, 13, 2-10.

Rogers, M. E. An introduction to the theoretical basis of nursing. Philadelphia: F. A. Davis, 1970.

Rosenblueth, A., & Wiener, N. The role of models in science. Philosophy of Science, 1945, 12, 316-321.

Roy, C., Sr. Adaptation: Implications for curriculum change. Nursing Outlook, 1973, 21, 163-168.

Roy, C., Sr. Introduction to nursing: An adaptation model. Englewood Cliffs, N.J.: Prentice-Hall, 1976.

Russell, C. S. Transition to parenthood: Problems and gratifica-
tions. Journal of Marriage and Family, 1974, 36, 294-301.

Sand, O. Curriculum study in basic nursing education. New York:
G. P. Putnam's Sons, 1955.

Sand, O. Editorial . . . Nursing education in the forefront. Nursing
Outlook, 1957, 5(1), 15.

Sand, O., & Belcher, H. C. An experience in basic nursing education. New York: G. P. Putnam's Sons, 1958.

Schlotfeldt, R. M. The need for a conceptual framework. In P. J.
Verhonick (Ed.), Nursing research I. Boston: Little, Brown
and Co., 1975.

Schwab, J. The concept of the structure of a discipline. The Educational Record, 1962, 43(3), 197-205.

Schwab, J. Structure of the disciplines: Meanings and significances.
In G. W. Ford & L. Pugno (Eds.), The structure of knowledge
and the curriculum. Chicago: Rand McNally & Co., 1964.

Scriven, M. The methodology of evaluation. In Stalse, R. E. (Ed.),
Perspectives of curriculum evaluation, American Educational
Research Association Monograph Series on Evaluation No. 1.
Chicago: Rand McNally & Co., 1967.

Seguel, M. L. The curriculum field: Its formative years. New
York: Teacher's College Press, 1966.

Selltiz, C., Wrightsman, L. S., & Cook, S. W. Research methods
in social relations (3rd ed.). New York: Holt, Rinehart and
Winston, 1976.

Shamansky, S. L., & Clausen, C. L. Levels of prevention: Examination of the concept. Nursing Outlook, 1980, 28, 104-108.

Selye, H. The physiology and pathology of exposure to stress.
Montreal: ACTA, 1950.

Sheahan, M. On accreditation. The American Journal of Nursing,
1960, 60(10), 1475-1478.

Sidelaeau, B. Stress and the mind-body interrelationship. In
J. Haber et al. (Eds.), Comprehensive psychiatric nursing.
New York: McGraw-Hill, 1978.

Silva, M. C. Philosophy, science, theory: Interrelationships and
implications for nursing research. Image, 1977, 9, 59-63.

Smith, C. M. What sources and technics shall we use in revising
the curriculum? The American Journal of Nursing, 1935, 35,
459-465.

Spanier, G. B. Measuring dyadic adjustment: New scales for assessing the quality of marriage and similar dyads. Journal of Marriage and the Family, 1976, 38, 15-28.

Steele, J. M. Dimensions of the class activities questionnaire. Illinois Gifted Program and Center for Instructional Research and Curriculum Evaluation, University of Illinois, 1969.

Stevens, B. J. Analysis of structural forms used in nursing curricula. Nursing Research, 1971, 20(5), 388-397.

Stevens, B. J. Nursing theory. Boston: Little, Brown and Co., 1979.

Stewart, I. M. The education of nurses. New York: Macmillan Co., 1943.

Stewart, I. M. What educational philosophy shall we accept for the new curriculum? The American Journal of Nursing, 1935, 35, 259-267.

Strauss, A. The structure of ideology of American nursing: An Interpretation. In F. Davis (Ed.), The nursing profession: Five sociological essays. New York: John Wiley & Sons, 1966.

Stuckly, D. J., & Cook, E. E. Are elective pass/fail grading systems compatible with the concept of academic excellence? Journal of Agronomic Education, 1976, 5, 57-60.

Styles, M. In the name of integration. Nursing Outlook, 1976, 24(12), 738-744.

Taba, H. Curriculum development. New York: Harcourt, Brace & World, 1962.

Tanner, D., & Tanner, L. Curriculum development. New York: Macmillan Co., 1975.

Taylor, A. L., & Mandrillo, M. P. A survey and analysis of bachelor degree recipients from the School of Nursing of the University of Virginia, 1969-1972. Charlottesville, Va.: Office of Instructional Analysis, 1973.

Taylor, E. J. The next step forward. The American Journal of Nursing, 1935, 35, 57-58.

Thibodeau, J. Adult performance on cognitive development tests as a function of task content, career level and cognitive style. Unpublished doctoral dissertation, University of Massachusetts, 1978.

Torres, G. Educational trends and the integrated curriculum approach in nursing. In Faculty-curriculum development, part IV, Unifying the curriculum—The integrated approach. New York: National League for Nursing, 1974.

Torres, G., & Yura, H. The meaning and functions of concepts and theories within education and nursing. In Faculty-curriculum development, part III, Conceptual framework—Its meaning and function. New York: National League for Nursing, 1975.

Tschudin, M. S., Belcher, H. C., & Nedelsky, L. Evaluation in basic nursing education. New York: G. P. Putnam's Sons, 1958.

Tung, D. A. Parenthood as crisis and related factors. Unpublished term paper. Storrs, Conn.: University of Connecticut School of Nursing, 1977.

Tyler, R. W. Basic principles of curriculum and instruction. Chicago: The University of Chicago Press, 1949.

University of Connecticut School of Nursing. Curriculum project report, academic year 1973-1974. Unpublished report. Storrs, Conn.: University of Connecticut School of Nursing, 1974.

University of Connecticut School of Nursing. Curriculum project report, academic year 1974-1975. Unpublished report. Storrs, Conn.: University of Connecticut School of Nursing, 1975.

University of Connecticut School of Nursing. Final report of the five year curriculum project. Unpublished report. Storrs, Conn.: University of Connecticut School of Nursing, July 1977.

Vaillot, M. C. Nursing theory, levels of nursing, and curriculum development. Nursing Forum, 1970, 9, 234-249.

Walsh, M. Why nursing education programs should be accredited. New York: National League for Nursing, 1975.

Weiner, G. The interaction among anxiety, stress instructions, and difficulty. Journal of Consulting Psychology, 1959, 23, 324-328.

White, M., & Coburn, D. The trials, tribulations, and tensions of curriculum change. Nursing Outlook, 1977, 25, 644-649.

Williams, C. A. The nature and development of conceptual frameworks. In F. S. Downs & J. W. Fleming (Eds.), Issues in nursing research. New York: Appleton-Century-Crofts, 1979.

Windwer, C. Relationship among prospective parents' locus of control, social desirability, and choice of psychoprophylaxis. Nursing Research, 1977, 26, 96-99.

Wolf-Wilets, V., & Nugent, L. C. A political analysis of curriculum change. Nursing Outlook, 1979, 27, 207-211.

Wu, R. R. Designing a curriculum model. Journal of Nursing Education, 1979, 18(3), 13-21.

Yura, H., & Torres, G. Today's conceptual frameworks within baccalaureate nursing programs. In Faculty-curriculum development, part III, Conceptual framework—Its meaning and function. New York: National League for Nursing, 1975.

Zbilut, J. P. Epistemologic constraints to the development of a theory of nursing (Letter to the Editor). Nursing Research, 1978, 27, 128-129.

Index